ABOUT THE AUTHOR

Alice Jolly is a novelist, playwright and teacher of creative writing. Her two novels (*What the Eye Doesn't See* and *If Only You Knew*) are both published by Simon and Schuster. She is completing a third novel. Her articles have been published in the *Guardian*, the *Mail on Sunday* and the *Independent* and she has broadcast on Radio 4. Four of her plays have been professionally produced by The Everyman Theatre in Cheltenham. Two of these plays were funded by The Arts Council. Her monologues have been performed in London and provincial theatres and she has recently been commissioned by Paines Plough ('The National Theatre of New Writing'). In 2014 one of her short stories won the V. S. Pritchett Memorial Prize awarded by The Royal Society of Literature. She teaches for The Arvon Foundation and on the Oxford University Master's Degree in Creative Writing. She has lived in Warsaw and in Brussels. She has three children – a son who is twelve, a daughter who was stillborn and a daughter who was born to a surrogate mother in the United States. Her home is now in Stroud in Gloucestershire and she is married to Stephen Kinsella.

DEAD BABIES

AND

SEASIDE TOWNS

Alice Jolly

unbound

First published in 2015 by Unbound

This edition published in 2017

Unbound
6th Floor Mutual House, 70 Conduit Street, London W1S 2GF
www.unbound.co.uk

Typeset by Bracketpress

Grateful acknowledgements to:
The Provost and Scholars of King's College, Cambridge and
The Society of Authors and the E. M. Forster Estate

Excerpt from *No Author Better Served: The Correspondence of Samuel Beckett and Alan Schneider*. Copyright © 2000 by Harvard University Press. All rights reserved.

Excerpt(s) from *Traveling Mercies: Some Thoughts on Faith* by Anne Lamott, copyright © 1999 by Anne Lamott. Used by permission of Pantheon Books, an imprint of the Knopf Doubleday Publishing Group, a division of Penguin Random House LLC. All rights reserved.

Excerpt from *The Second Four Books of Poems* by W. S. Merwin, copyright © 1993 by W. S. Merwin. Used by permission of Copper Canyon Press and The Wylie Agency. All rights reserved.

Art direction by Mecob

A CIP record for this book
is available from the British Library

ISBN 978-1-78352-105-0 (trade hbk)
ISBN 978-1-78352-160-9 (ebook)
ISBN 978-1-78352-106-7 (limited edition)
ISBN 978-1-78352-361-0 (paperback)

Printed in Great Britain by Clays Ltd, St Ives Plc

1 3 5 7 9 8 6 4 2

To Stephen Kinsella –

Always a springboard and a soft landing.

Photo acknowledgements:
Photo of Hope – Louise Buckley
Photo of Hope and Thomas – John Lawrence
Moniack Mhor – Nancy MacDonald
Five Naked Ladies – Joslin Towler
The Falling Lady – Rose Towler
The Grand, Brighton
whatisbelgium.blogspot.be
Helen Sargeant

ACKNOWLEDGEMENTS

My thanks first and foremost to all who subscribed to this book. Without you, the book would not have been been published. I would also like to thank: Clare Andrews, Kathleen Jones, Susannah Rickards, Xandra Bingley, Amanda Holmes Duffy, Isabel Costello, Katie Waldegrave, Gillian Stern, Caroline Sanderson, Paola Schweitzer, Samantha Caswell, John Boyle, Jeannette Cook, Loretta Stanley, Martin Westlake, Katie Beringer, Linda McKinnon, Polly Rendell, Christa Mahana, Sally Frapwell, Jo Lowde, Lyndall Gibson, Catherine Large, Joanna O'Malley, Clare Dunkel, Mandy Fenton, everyone at The Quaker Meeting Houses in Brussels and Nailsworth, my friends at The Everyman Theatre in Cheltenham, Dr Clare Morgan and all my colleagues and students on the Oxford Masters' Degree in Creative Writing, Victoria Hobbs at A.M. Heath and, in particular, John Mitchinson, Isobel Frankish, Lauren Fulbright and all their colleagues at Unbound.

I

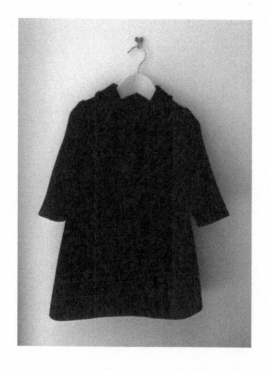

Your absence has gone through me
like thread through a needle.
Everything I do is stitched with its color.

W. S. Merwin – 'Separation'

I see Laura often, running in a frost-glittered garden. She is two years old, a tiny flame-flicker of a child, just as her older brother Thomas was at that age. She wears a navy blue beret and her silver-blonde hair is cut bluntly and falls to just above her shoulders. Her blue wool coat is fitted at the waist and has a rounded velvet collar and large velvet-covered buttons. The frost has made her skin blue-white, her lips a smear of red, a wound that will not heal.

She dashes past me at such speed that my image of her is blurred – an arm stretched forward, both feet in their T-bar, navy shoes suspended above the ground. Her legs are thin as wire and her woollen tights wrinkle at the ankle. The toe of that stretched-forward foot is pulled back towards her shin. Somewhere out of sight, other children are running as well, chasing each other, ducking and swivelling, their laughter crackling in the brittle air.

But where is she? In the garden at Mount Vernon. I know that – but where exactly? Behind her a flower bed is thick with scarlet roses which bloom despite the frost. I feel sure that she's on the lawn, just below the coach house hedge, but no child could run on such steep ground. Other children will grow up, change, disappoint, amaze, but not Laura. Even if I live to be one hundred, she will still be running – endlessly running – past the winter roses in her navy blue beret.

It began in a house in North London, one of those toppling, red-brick terraced houses, stacked up tight against each other in the streets above Gospel Oak. We were staying with friends for the weekend and that morning we walked to a playground on the edge of Hampstead Heath. My husband, Stephen, pushed our son, two-year-old Thomas, on swings and stood beside metal-runged ladders, guiding wavering, wellington-booted feet.

It was warm for March and yet I sat on a bench shivering in two jumpers, a coat, scarves, boots and gloves. I was nearly three months pregnant with our second child. My stomach rolled and heaved, my lips were dry, my mouth tasted sour and even the wind on my face felt like an assault. I longed for time to sweep me on, past twelve weeks of pregnancy, as I knew that then the sandpaper-rawness and nagging sickness might end.

After we came back from the Heath, our friends Mark and Susan cooked us a proper Sunday lunch – lamb, roast potatoes, buttery cabbage – which we ate amidst the half-finished building work in their kitchen. I pushed down two plates despite the nausea. A taxi had been called to take us to the Eurostar at Waterloo Station. From there we would travel back to our home in Brussels.

As we cleared the table, Mark and Susan's three children and Thomas were scurrying through the house, their feet clattering, their voices shrieking, determined to fall over the tins of paint left by the builders, smash their heads against the piles of floorboards stacked in the hall, or fall down the uncarpeted stairs. I went to help Stephen with the pushchair and the bags, then hurried to the loo – and that's when I found the warning stain of blood.

I mentioned it to Susan. Neither of us knew what to do. Susan said she'd bled once with one of her three and went to find a sanitary towel. Bizarrely it was wrapped in orange plastic and, as Susan is an artist who often works with bright colours, the idea entered my mind that she had made it. Stephen was uncertain whether we should get into the taxi or not but we set off for Waterloo. As the taxi stop-started through Kentish Town and lurched through Camden, I thought – *So this is it then, I'm going to lose this baby after eleven weeks of pregnancy*. But my mind did not accept that possibility. And it turned out that I didn't need to worry because, by the time we were on the train, the bleeding had stopped.

Later – much later – when I thought back to that Gospel Oak house, what I remembered was the shrieks of the children as they scurried on the stairs and the sunlight shining in through the Georgian fanlight above the front door, making a pattern of blue, yellow and red lozenges on the tiled floor. Also the orange plastic package of that sanitary towel, which I never used, and still have, upstairs in the bathroom cupboard.

Although I'm a writer by profession, I have always felt sure that I would never write a memoir. I do not trust them, never have. Me-me-me, moi-moi-moi. But now our legal team – one law firm in America, two law firms in England and a barrister – have been in touch to say that I need to write a twenty-page statement explaining everything that happened. They need this in preparation for our hearing in the High Court.

And so I go to my study and pull out the cardboard box which contains the last five years of my life. A ragged pile of diaries, photos, e-mails, blog entries, sentences scrawled in notebooks. But how can I organise it? My mind is fuzzy, my neck and shoulders are sore and even opening the box makes my throat close up. I really have no idea how the jigsaw of days and months fits together. It isn't just the years which have gone but the person who occupied them as well.

Keep hold of the facts. There must be some. I am now forty-five but I used to be younger. A good friend tells me that if I were ever to write a memoir it would be called *The Spectre at the Feast*. I frequently forget that the over-examined life isn't worth living. As we don't have a television, my views are supplied by *The Guardian* and Radio 4 and consequently I am both meticulously well informed and appallingly out of touch. My husband describes me as having no post-Brontë cultural references. My family refer to me as All Brains and No Sense. I am in love with R.S. Thomas, a poet who is cantankerous, dead and Welsh. And even more in love with seaside towns.

And after that? There are no other facts – only days. Days which begin with a sudden shock, as though I'm new from the womb. Here we are. Still alive. Miraculously, outrageously, still here. And the dear old sun performing that wonderfully clever trick again, sliding up over the horizon, as I bundle Thomas, nine years old now, yawning, with a bag full of football kit, into the car. And set off across Rodborough Common, through the frost-silent morning, with nothing holding the whole thing together except sinew and bone.

Why look at the contents of that box? Why try to reassemble the fractured fragments into something new? So much better to focus on that vast orange ball of the dawn sun as it emerges from the mist, better to enjoy the silhouettes of trees on the horizon like intricate black lace. Sinew and bone. Nothing else. How strange to discover how much I enjoy my non-existent existence.

But now – in this endless period of waiting – the lawyer e-mails again demanding that twenty-page document. So I pull out that box once more. Breathe, remember to breathe. Wedding anniversaries? Might that be the way to sort things out? When Stephen and I got married, we decided that we would celebrate each anniversary by visiting places in alphabetical order. For example, the first year would be Antibes, the second Bali, the third the Canaries. And after that Dubai, Egypt, Fuerteventura and Ghana.

But I got pregnant with Thomas straight after our wedding and so our anniversaries became a tour of the Brussels suburbs – Anderlecht, Boitsfort, and then the Place du Châtelain, the square at the end of our road. Then D for death and after that – Eastbourne. I do remember Eastbourne, the comfort of the sea mist, tea from one of those metal service-station pots which don't pour properly, and somewhere in the distance Beachy Head, with the pale green sea heaving in.

But after that the reception scrambles, the sound crackles and falters, the lines on the screen break up into fuzzing black and white zigzags. It's like when you play the piano and your left hand stretches down to a low note, a distant C, but it doesn't make the sound that it should. Instead the thread of your melody breaks up in a discordant clanking. And then you notice that the lower section of the keyboard is upside down and back to front, the familiar pattern of black and white all jumbled up. Where there should be a C there is now an F or a G.

When you write a novel you work with chains of cause and effect, moments of resolution where meaning might briefly and brilliantly dazzle through. Will it be the same if I write a memoir? No. I wouldn't dare now to hope for so much. I aim merely to establish the chronology. I want only to stretch my mind back through the past and find the notes of my keyboard where they should properly be. Recently I went back to that North London house and there is no stained glass fanlight above the front door.

II

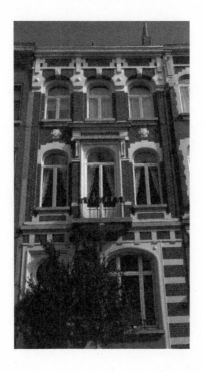

We have art in order not to die of the truth.

Friedrich Nietzche

Later – much later – when I went to a support group meeting, the lady running the session asked us all to think of the moment before it happened, the moment when our dreams were about to turn to nightmare. She suggested that we should all bring along a photograph of that moment to the next meeting. I couldn't see the point and don't have a photograph.

But I do have a memory – a vivid memory. It was 2005, the weekend before Easter – two weeks after Hampstead Heath – and Stephen, Thomas and I had travelled back to England from our home in Brussels to spend a few days with family in Gloucestershire. And as my mum had offered to look after Thomas, I was free, gloriously, spectacularly free. After three months of morning sickness, I was basking in the simple pleasure of feeling well.

And so I drove from my mum's farm in Worcestershire to Hay-on-Wye and spent the day with our friend Matthew. The air tasted fresh and sharp as lemon juice and everywhere was brimming full of vivid green. Matthew and I bought sandwiches and sat together on the castle wall and talked, as we do talk, about all the big stuff. God and death and whether it all means anything.

But it wasn't the words that mattered. Instead what I remember is the sense of height – dizzying, spinning height – as we perched up on the castle walls. And the view of the hills opposite – grey-green and vast – rearing up in front of us into the dull haze of the spring sky. And far away on one of those distant slopes, suspended up near the clouds, a farmhouse and barns, surrounded by a jigsaw of stone walls, their colours merging into the shades of the land. Yes, the farm on the hills above Hay-on-Wye. The last of innocence.

The third day of April 2005 – I don't need to search through my cardboard box to verify that date. A month after that North London weekend, two weeks after the farm on the hill. And I wake up to find that the bleeding has started again. I am sixteen weeks pregnant. Thomas is on the landing sitting in his laundry basket ship, taking his teddies on a voyage to Australia.

I whisper to Stephen, then go downstairs to ring the hospital. They tell me to come in for a scan and so Stephen rings his office to cancel a meeting and I coax Thomas out of the laundry basket. Then we drive him to nursery in our second-hand Peugeot 106 and head on to the Hospital of St Clare, two miles from our house, in the Brussels suburb of Uccle. Every few minutes the muscles in my lower back contract and I clench my teeth against the pain.

St Clare is a modern hospital, gleaming white with huge sun-filled windows. I go to the reception desk of the Gynaecology Department and, speaking in French, explain. The receptionist makes a call and says things I don't understand. We are told to sit down and wait. There is no waiting room, just a circular, windowless bulge in the corridor, lined by wooden slatted seats. A doctor I don't know arrives and asks questions. My ability to speak French evaporates. As I stumble through my story, I feel the other waiting women shift, fold themselves away. A clearness of air, a silence, emerges around me even in that crowded space. A nurse arrives with a wheelchair and tells me to sit in it. I don't feel ill enough for a wheelchair but I do what I'm told.

There seems to be some delay with the appointments. People shrug and sigh. *Mais pourquoi? Quel est le problème? Que se passe-t-il ici?* Apparently there's an emergency so some routine appointments will have to wait. Stephen and I nod at each other. We are polite and reasonable people, the kind of people who almost relish an opportunity to stand aside and let some other more needy person take our place. Another doctor emerges, peers at me, disappears.

Then I understand. I am the emergency.

Finally I am wheeled into the cramped, windowless office occupied by Dr Vermeulen. She is a tiny, boyish Flemish woman of no particular age. Her eyes are round as pennies and glitter blue in an elfin face. She looks fragile but I remember that, when she delivered Thomas, she stripped down to a singlet and revealed herself to be pure muscle. Her English is immaculate and she is well known among the British in Brussels.

She takes me through to another cramped room across the corridor. This is where they do the scans. The blind at the window is pulled down. I take off the bottom half of my clothing. Stephen sits on a chair in the corner beside a folded screen. The lights go down and Dr Vermeulen spreads cold, blue jelly across my abdomen. We see our baby on the screen and immediately we hear a rushing throb, then a hurried thump, thump, thump.

Dr Vermeulen moves the sensor and watches the screen in front of her.

Something is going on here, she says. Yes, the placenta is partly detached.

Is it serious? I ask.

Yes, she says.

I wait for her to qualify this but she is silent.

This is too early, she says. This is much too early.

Then she makes a tutting sound and sighs.

The placenta is too low, she says. A part of it has become detached. It may fail at any time. It's a rare condition this, and dangerous. It's possible for the baby to survive on only two thirds of the placenta but you are at serious risk of infection.

I wait but she says nothing more.

And the baby?

The baby may live – or die. It just isn't possible to say.

There's nothing you can do? Stephen asks.

No. Nothing. You just have to wait. You might be lucky and you might not. She sighs again, shakes her head. I just hope you don't get to six or seven months of this pregnancy and lose this baby, she says. That's something I wouldn't wish on anyone. The only thing you can do is to try not to move too much. There's no scientific evidence that this will help – but it's worth a try.

As I put my clothes back on, I'm strangely calm. Stephen and I leave the Gynaecology Department, walk back through the sun-bright corridors, past the pneumatic doors of the Paediatrics Department and a room with a children's play-house. I move carefully, trying not to jerk a single muscle. I am running an egg and spoon race, blindfolded. I must keep the egg on the spoon but I don't know if I'm succeeding. Our baby might die and I won't even know. Stephen and I agree that we're going to fight for the life of our baby – but the only way we can fight is if I lie down.

At home I take up residence on the sofa and try not to move but our house is a classic Belgian town house – toweringly tall and thin – with more than ninety stairs. And everything I need is on another floor. Small decisions become momentous. I've finished my book and I want to start another but it's downstairs. Shall I go and fetch it? Or will that kill my baby? This is the paradox: I am totally responsible for the safety of this baby but the whole situation is far beyond my control.

Over the next week, the bleeding doesn't stop but it doesn't get worse. The hospital have given me endless pills to take and they numb the worst of the pain. We have no family in Brussels but Stephen has just left his law firm and has been put on paid gardening leave, for a whole year. Friends refer to him as The Constant Gardener. We don't feel in the mood to share the joke but this is a stroke of luck, as it allows him to take over the day-to-day work of the house. We are together often but we don't say much. I am close to finishing my second novel so I try to write with my laptop on my knee but the angle is awkward, and I can't concentrate, so I give up and read R.S. Thomas's poems instead.

I invent an awkward acronym in my head – NRTIHRN. Nothing Really Terrible Is Happening Right Now. And it's true. Right now, in these particular spring days, the world is luminous and gentle. The sofa I occupy is in our first floor sitting room, a room decorated all in blue with three long windows looking out over the street. From the sofa I can see the blackened red brick of the houses opposite, their curving Art Nouveau window frames and iron balconies. Every hour the bells ring out from the convent in the next street. Occasionally a car passes but, other than that, silence. In this house it's always impossible to believe that we're a mile from the centre of a capital city.

Sometimes I move upstairs to the guest room. From there, propped against pillows, I can see the trees in other gardens, the red roofs of distant houses. The white of apple blossom is sharp against the new green around it. Sadly I'm not at the right angle to see our garden but Stephen tells me that our plum tree is thick with blossom too. I think of summers when that tree has been heavy with fruit and how we've brought it all down with a ladder and sticks, and taken the plums out into the street for the neighbours to share.

At the weekends, Stephen puts a camp bed downstairs in the breakfast room so that I can watch Thomas play, or chat to the occasional friends who bring their children around for tea. I have the sense that these friends believe that I am engaged in some extreme form of hypochondria. They all tell stories of other women they know who have bled during pregnancy. *You know she lost four pints. She lost six, eight. But still she finished up with a perfectly healthy baby in the end.* So no need to worry.

These friends also find it difficult to accept that the medical profession can do nothing. I am urged to try a different doctor, a different hospital. It seems that it's hard for the modern mind to accept that there are limits to what technology can do. We all watch every detail of a pregnancy developing on a screen but we're seldom faced with the realisation that, when a pregnancy goes wrong, there's nothing that the medical profession can do, except watch.

We have been told that we should go back to the hospital every two weeks. Those appointments provide the structure of our days. It's five days to the next appointment, four days, three, two, one. I've been lying flat on my back for four weeks now and so when appointment day arrives I'm as excited as a child off on a school trip. I dress carefully, put on make-up, a white T-shirt, a loose black dress and my favourite lilac scarf. I refuse to be pitiful. Dr Vermeulen does a scan and tells us that the situation is no better and no worse. We ask what sex the baby is because we're longing for a little girl but Dr Vermeulen avoids our question.

After the appointment, with Dr Vermeulen's approval, Stephen and I risk a coffee in the hospital café. Two heavily pregnant women talk at the next table. For them, pregnancy is fluffy wool blankets, and new buggies and mobiles made up of wooden clouds and rainbows. One wants a water birth.

The other is hoping for a boy but doesn't want to find out in advance. I feel like shouting – *Don't you know? Don't you understand? It isn't like that at all.* But then I take hold of my mind and realise that I'm glad that they don't know. I want them never to have to know.

In the car, going home from the hospital, my eyes eat up the details of the streets as they pass. The Brasserie St Georges at the entrance to Avenue Winston Churchill, where waiters in full livery appear on the terraces and serve vast platters of oysters, *moules*, *frites*, mayonnaise. The yellow and blue trams passing the Bois de la Cambre. The gentle spring wind catching at the leaves of trees, a stray plastic bag dancing through warm air. And the people with the normal lives, striding past the shopping centre on the Chaussée de Vleurgat, heading out to buy a *sandwich américain* or meet a friend for lunch.

It seems so strange that these people don't know the luxury they enjoy, don't appreciate the gift of walking in the street, lunching with a friend. I want to wind down the car window and call out to them, remind them to enjoy the fresh air, the trams passing, the lunchtime sandwich, as much as they can. As the car moves on, I promise myself that once I'm able to move again then I will wring enjoyment out of every tiny thing. But even as I make that promise, I know that the world doesn't work like that.

Two-year-old Thomas knows that Mummy is ill and mustn't get up from the sofa but still he climbs onto me, very gently. I tell him that it's all right for him to sit on my legs but not my tummy. He pats his tiny hand on my thigh – Is this your tummy? Can I sit here? Or here?

But one evening Stephen is out and Thomas refuses to go to bed. I speak to him firmly but he is stubborn. Usually I would take hold of him and carry him, wailing and kicking, up the stairs, but I don't dare lift him. Finally I burst into tears and he weeps as well. Then he takes my hand and leads me upstairs and we lie in bed together, while I pretend that I'm not crying. He brings me a teddy from his toy box and gives it to me to cuddle.

Cuddling a teddy is a good way to feel better, he tells me.

Then he brings more and more cuddly toys, piling them all around the bed, so that by the time that he snuggles in next to me, we've got teddies crammed in all around us. Mungo, Alfie, Purdey, Red Nose Moose, The Selfish Crocodile and Peter Rabbit. The whole toy box full. Together we get the giggles, smothered beneath the piles of furry animals.

One of Thomas's favourite games is to sit in the laundry basket with those same teddies and sail around the world, visiting a random selection of real cities, fairy-tale locations, grandmothers and cousins. One morning, I lie in bed and watch him sail his ship as Stephen shaves. His hair is silver and gold, his long dark lashes sweep down across his cheeks in a delicate fan, and his face is entirely serious, lost in the adventure of the laundry basket ship and its cargo of furry passengers.

So where are you going in your ship? I ask.

He gives me a withering look. Mummy, it's not a ship. It's a laundry basket.

You better watch out, Stephen says. He'll be calling the Social Services and complaining that his mother doesn't know the difference between a laundry basket and a ship.

I laugh – but carefully because otherwise the pain might start – and watch Thomas trying to get something down from a shelf. He can't reach it and now Stephen has gone downstairs to make some tea. The shelves are high and heavy, Thomas is wobbling on the bottom shelf, stretching his hand up and pulling at a jigsaw above. I imagine the shelves toppling, falling, crashing down onto his tiny, fragile bones. And so I start to lower my legs to the floor.

As I move, some minute valve opens inside me. And suddenly I'm soaked in blood. *This is it*, I think. *Our baby has died.* But the bleeding stops as suddenly as it came. I keep silent, hoping that Thomas won't turn around. Stephen appears, sees the blood, lifts Thomas down from the shelves and sweeps him out of the room, inventing a story about a cat in the garden. I start to clear up the mess and wonder whether I should go to hospital but they've told me there's no point unless the bleeding is serious. But what is serious? Finally I do nothing because I know that the hospital can't help. Stephen doesn't manage to clear up everything before he has to leave. The bloodstained sheets lie on top of the laundry basket all day because I don't dare take them down to the washing machine.

After that I become paranoid about blood. A pool of tomato sauce left on the side of a plate glares angry and red. Even though I shouldn't move, I put the plate in the dishwasher. Stains of red wine on the kitchen table are ominous. I need to get a grip but I can't. My nose bleeds and I panic before I remember that a baby can't die because of a nosebleed. A child comes around to the house and holds a tipping cup of Cherryade. I scream at Stephen to get hold of the cup because if that red liquid spills then our baby will die. Just keep all the red liquid in bottles or cups and we will all survive.

I begin to feel our baby move. Friends tell me that I must be mistaken, it's too early, but I know they're wrong. The feeling is like tiny fingers fluttering against the inside of my skin. I lie in bed with my hand pressed against my belly, waiting for that feeling, imagining our baby, so close, just under my skin, his or her hand touching mine.

The bleeding is no worse. Ten days to the next hospital appointment. Nine, eight, seven. Thomas has started wetting the bed. I'm worried about my unfinished novel. I've already missed the deadline by a whole year but I am close to finishing. How will that ever happen now? Our brief and brilliant spring has come to an end. The weather is cold and rainy and the blossom is falling. When I move down to the breakfast room at the weekend, I see it piled up on the terrace, slowly turning brown. Presumably we will have no plums this year?

One night, lying in bed, I hear a loud and rhythmic banging coming from next door. It echoes through the walls of the house and thumps inside my head. It seems odd that our neighbours should start doing building work late at night – and what are they doing which involves this loud and regular hammering? Stephen comes up to bed and I mention that the noise is keeping me awake. He tells me that there is no noise. And I realise that what I'm hearing is my own fear.

III

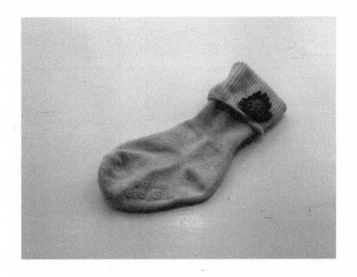

A person's fears are lighter when
the danger is at hand.

Seneca

Chronology. I get the diaries out of the cardboard box and check. I know exactly what happened but my mind muddles the sequence of events. People think that you become a writer because you have knowledge that other people don't possess. In fact, the opposite is true. Most writers – whether professional or amateur – write because they're trying to recover some knowledge which was part of their birthright, but which was lost to them far back in time, right at the beginning.

All the non-writing people have this knowledge, without even knowing they have it. To them, it's as obvious as breathing. But the writer goes through agonies, struggles with the blank page, covers three hundred sheets of paper, only to discover that he or she has brought to birth some brief glimpse of a widely accepted truth. So it is that my main feeling about writers – myself included – is one of pity. Like the low grade magician at a children's party who, with a bold flourish, finally produces the rabbit from the hat, only to be humiliated by the merciless small boy at the front of the assembled crowd who announces loudly – *I saw him, I saw him. He had it up his sleeve all the time.*

Three days to the next hospital appointment. It's morning and Stephen has already taken Thomas to nursery and is now getting ready to go to Paris for the day. I lean over to pick up my book and the bleeding comes again in a massive flood. I stand up in an attempt to save the bedclothes and buckets of scarlet liquid spread across the white floorboards. My eyes flick away, up to the skylight above – grey-blue sky, the dirty edge of a cloud. I try to draw breath but no air will enter my lungs. *So this is it then. Our baby has died.* Stephen heads for the telephone and starts to ring the hospital. I stare at the pool of red on the floor. But then I feel small feet kicking inside me, firm and true. *I'm all right, Mummy. I'm all right. And so are you. Yes, you are.*

In the Casualty department, I expect alarms to ring, stretchers to appear. But instead I'm sent up to the maternity ward where I'm unable to establish who can help. Eventually I'm shown into a delivery room. It may even be the same room in which Thomas was born nearly three years ago. I find the technology in the hospital comforting. I feel sure that, even though they've said there's nothing they can do, still they will find some way of helping me. They do a scan and say that the baby is fine. I begin to feel more confident. I'm borrowing my courage from our baby now. If this hasn't killed him, or her, then nothing will.

I spend all day at the hospital, alone in the delivery room, feeling our baby's feather fingers stroking and fluttering inside me. The hospital seems oddly quiet. The view from the window is the suburbs of Brussels – a tower block, a kite caught in a tree, looping telephone wires, satellite dishes barnacled on every house. Six weeks have passed since the bleeding started and I'm now twenty weeks pregnant. All I have to do is keep getting through the days. NRTIHRN. I wrap myself up in my purple wool shawl. All day I hear women in other delivery rooms giving birth.

I'm sorry, one of the nurses said. It does get rather noisy.

But it isn't the women in pain which bothers me, it's the cries of the babies. That strange anguished haunting cry, so full of grief, which is like no other sound.

I'm now twenty-two weeks pregnant. Every time I stand up, the floor is covered with blood. I'm admitted to hospital. Both Stephen and I are relieved because doubtless in the Hospital of St Clare – with its shiny plate-glass windows and stacks of technology – all will be well. Nothing as old-fashioned and vulgar as death could happen there. In my head, I run endless calculations. Twenty-four weeks is the earliest they can deliver a baby. So I just need to keep the egg on the spoon for two more weeks. We'll get there, I know we will.

From my hospital bed, there's no view, only sky. Unless I push a knob to raise the bed and then I can glimpse washing on a roof terrace, a jumble of red tiled roofs, skylights and chimneys. A new wing is being built onto the hospital and from outside the noise of construction work is continual. Diggers grind and clank, pneumatic drills rattle, scaffolding poles clatter. I can't wash my hair or shave my legs. At first the nurses allow me to get out of bed to go to the loo but after a while I'm not even allowed to do that. The bleeding doesn't stop but every few hours they put a strap over my belly and I can hear the baby's heart.

The days consist of endless blood-soaked sanitary towels that the nurses come to examine. Sometimes the catheter in my arm doesn't work properly and the nurses have to move it. My veins, they tell me, are deceptive. They're easy to see but when they try to put a needle in them they roll. Sometimes when they have to move the catheter it takes them four attempts to pierce a vein, and they finish up digging into old bruises. My arms are soon purple and black. I develop a rash which starts on my feet and spreads all over my body. It itches until I want to tear my flesh from my bones. I read R. S. Thomas again and again, feel the calm of his poems seeping through me.

High up on the wall a television is set on a stand with a video underneath it. The clock on the television tells the correct time but the video clock is one hour slow. I play a game with myself, looking at the video clock first, then allowing my eyes to move up to the television, and savouring the joy of finding myself one hour further on. I'm told that, if I can get to twenty-four weeks, then I'll be moved to the Hospital of St Luke, which is a university hospital with specialist facilities for premature babies. Images of St Luke's flicker in and out of my mind, a distant dream, a mirage. Not long and I'll be there.

There are moments of happiness – books, phone calls, a television programme about Renaissance art in Italy, a patch of golden sunlight which settles on the wall opposite me in the evening. I spend hours on the telephone, calling Matthew in Hay-on-Wye and my friend Amanda, who used to live in Brussels, but now lives in Rome. Local friends come as well and my mum and my sister call several times a day. Mum longs to come to Brussels but is in bed with flu. But still NRTIHRN.

Outside my room the normal workings of a maternity ward are continuing but the nurses keep my door closed. One day a woman arrives from a florist with a bunch of flowers sent by a friend. She walks into the room with a broad smile on her face, obviously ready to congratulate me and admire my new baby. Then she sees the look on my face, dumps the flowers and runs.

My friend Rachel comes to the hospital with her two-year-old daughter Edie. Rachel is pregnant herself but her baby isn't due until November. She suggests knitting and, although I haven't knitted since I was a teenager, together we plan a scarf. She also brings a travel kettle, some builders' tea and fresh milk, a luxury in Brussels where nearly all milk is UHT.

After Rachel and Edie have left, a sock appears in the room – a little girl's sock, pink, with a blue flower stitched onto the cuff. I assume that this sock belongs to Edie, and has fallen out of Rachel's bag, but when Rachel comes again I ask her and she knows nothing of it. And so the sock stays where it is, lying on the table under the television.

Miranda comes as well, black-haired, brave Californian Miranda. She has troubles enough of her own. Her writer husband, Adam, has had shingles and it's left him with long-term health problems. And they have three small children. But she's still strong and full of confidence. I remember what Miranda looked like when I first met her, when Adam and she were newly married. She was beautiful then and she's still beautiful now but it's a different kind of beauty. We are none of us girls any more.

Thomas comes to the hospital with Big Alice, who is officially our Ghanaian cleaning lady, but is actually a grandmother to Thomas, and one of my best friends, despite the fact that I can only ever understand half of what she says. Thomas is fascinated by the lever that you can press to make the bed go up and down. He makes Big Alice push this again and again, shows me a picture he has made at nursery with pieces of pasta stuck on it, chases a balloon around the room, and then wants to go home.

A nurse tells me that she and the staff on the maternity ward are finding my situation difficult. We do not usually deal with problems of this kind, she says. It's not part of our job, we do not have the appropriate training. This is too serious and most upsetting for us. You should really be moved down to intensive care. Dr Vermeulen arrives and tells me that I should still expect to be in hospital for weeks, probably months.

I ask her if there is a danger that our baby will be born disabled.

No, she says. No. It won't happen like that. She will either live or die.

Strangely I am comforted. It helps that the situation is clear cut. I'm not a saint, I'm not even an averagely good person. If I had to bring up a badly disabled child then I suppose I would find the strength to do it but I'm essentially selfish and like my life as it is. It makes me feel guilty to realise this. But is Dr Vermeulen telling me the truth or just making a judgement about what I want to hear? I'm not sure. But I did notice the use of the word 'she'. So we are expecting a girl, just as we had hoped.

NRTIHRN. But the nights are difficult. I have so many hours in which to think. Me and my daughter, alone. Amanda in Rome, who has a more traditional faith than mine, quotes the Bible. *Yea though I walk through the valley of the shadow of death, I will fear no evil.* Somehow it helps to repeat those words. The clocks on the video and television pulse. Three in the morning. No, mercifully four. Only another hour until the light will come.

The problem is that I don't know where to position my mind. I should try to accept that our daughter might die. But if I do that then perhaps I am letting her down, bringing death closer by admitting that it might come? Usually it is always my policy to try to face up to the worst of any situation. Usually, once you've worked out what the worst thing that could happen is, you realise that it's not so very bad. But now that doesn't work because the worst is unimaginably bad.

I think of the last time I went to the sea, back in January, when I was newly pregnant. Stephen, Thomas and I went to a friend's fortieth birthday party in a massive grey stone house, surrounded by wind-battered peacocks, near Aberdovey, far out on the coast of West Wales. On the Sunday morning, after the party, Thomas woke appallingly early, as he often does, and so he and I were up alone in that hushed and shadowed house.

I felt sick and Thomas was whining so I bundled us both into coats and boots, put Thomas in the pushchair, and wheeled him through the waking peacocks, down the shaded, dawn lane, hoping that we might find the sea. The morning was sharp as glass, cold enough to make my nose run and my fingertips ache. As we walked, I thought of R. S. Thomas, because he'd lived only a few miles from Aberdovey and wrote nearly all of his poems about rural Wales, a place where he found no place to hide from God.

We walked for a long way together, Thomas and I, the pushchair bumping in the muddy lane. Until finally we came to a gate into a field cropped by sheep. And mysteriously, in the middle of this field, cut and pasted from another scene, was a train station. Just a stop on a single track line, a sign, a glass hut with a board showing a timetable. I didn't suppose this could be an operational train station but, as we drew closer, we saw the sign: Tonfanau. Thomas was delighted. He knows that I like trains and the sea so this was just the right place for us to be.

Fifty yards beyond the station was the sea. But there was no cliff, no beach – instead the field just dropped away over a sharp edge to the rolling waves below. In the early morning light, the place was desolate. Around us the hills – luminous green even at that time of year – rose up sharply. And suddenly I knew that we were not alone. This is a feeling I've had often before but now it was horribly intense.

The landscape pressed in on us. The hills were silently shouting. I thought of Munch and his tortured man on the bridge, not screaming himself, but overwhelmed by the scream of nature. This presence – whatever it was – had nothing to do with the God of light, lambs and love who I was taught about in my Church of England childhood. No wonder R.S. Thomas wrote here as he did.

Come on, I said. We've got to go.

And I hurried Thomas back across the field, trying not to feel that nameless presence which pressed in on us, trying not to see the accusing stare of the sky. But still I enjoyed my morning, and all the icy stillness and short-day greyness of that weekend. And I was glad that Thomas and our baby – so newly conceived – were there to share it with me.

But now in the Brussels hospital – at 4.30 in the morning – I ask what it was that I encountered that morning. A presence, or a force, something vast and limitless, something neither benevolent nor evil – but infinitely powerful. And is it that force which is in charge now? Which is making a decision about whether my baby will live or die? Of course not. It's all just random, it must be.

But I can't accept that whether my baby lives or dies will be decided by nothing more than the toss of a coin. So then who is in charge? And is it not possible for me to make a bargain with them? Given that I don't have any conventional religious belief, it would seem hypocritical to pray. And even if I did believe, wouldn't my prayers simply set God up for failure? But as the minutes tick on and the two clocks flash slowly through the darkness, I pray anyway because what else is there to do?

My baby may die. I need to stare into that vast expanse

of blackness, to know it for what it is. Was it Nietzsche who wanted to be able to say – *I want whatever happens*? No matter how hard I try, I can't say that. My mind baulks at taking the measure of this imagined loss. I call Matthew and then Amanda but neither of them picks up the phone. Who else can I talk to? Most of the people Stephen and I know in Brussels are people like us – affluent couples with professional jobs, comfortable houses, trouble-free children. They will only tell me yet more stories about the woman who lost two, four, six, eight pints of blood in pregnancy and yet finished up with a healthy baby.

But then, the next evening, I remember – the Quaker Meeting House. I am not a Quaker and I don't go to the Meeting House often but I have a great respect for the Quakers. I like their reticent, meticulous lives, their lack of any fixed creed, their scrupulous insistence that no one person should interfere in the spiritual life of another. I know that if I ask any of the Quakers a direct question then I will at least get a direct answer.

It's late when this thought comes to me but still I telephone Samuel Haydn who is the Clerk of the Meeting House. He's in his seventies, an American who has lived in Belgium all his life – a stocky man with bright eyes, a big beard and startling vigour. I know that he has a grown-up son who had a brain tumour as a child – and that the operation to remove it left him permanently damaged. He now has a part-time job in the local library in Anderlecht but Samuel and his wife worry about who will look after him when they're gone.

Samuel listens to my story and assures me that everyone at the Meeting will 'hold me in the light'. He uses those words because Quakers are wary of talk about prayer. But right now I need to talk about prayer and so we do, with no preamble. This elderly man whom I do not know talks about prayer as other people talk about traffic jams or gardening projects. I lie on the white hospital sheets with a blanket pulled over me and the phone pressed to my ear. The reading light above my bed wraps me in a sphere of light.

There is only one prayer which is important, Samuel says. And that is the prayer which asks that, whatever the outcome is, we shall find the strength to bear it with equanimity. He quotes William Littleboy – *We pray, not to change God's will, but to bring our wills into correspondence with His.*

Yes, I say. Yes. I know. But it doesn't work. Because I simply cannot make myself believe that our baby could die.

Ah yes, I see, Samuel says. Yes. I think in your particular circumstance it wouldn't work. How can one face the death of a baby with equanimity? No one can do that. No one should.

I wait for him to say something else but he doesn't. Silence is the Quaker gift and a man like Samuel knows when there is nothing more to be said. After I put the phone down I feel something of his particular silence, and the peace of the Meeting House, remaining in the room.

Only a few more days and I'll be up to twenty-four weeks. Then I'll be moved to St Luke's and they might be able to deliver our daughter. I don't care that she will be very premature. I know how strong she is because I can feel her kicking. I don't doubt that she'll make it through. But then, late one evening, I start shaking convulsively, my body jumping up and down off the bed. The nurses run to make a hot water bottle and tea. They tell me that this is a panic attack. Because my sister suffers from panic attacks, I'm able to believe that maybe this is just a trick of my mind, the fear of fear. But the nurses are wrong. It isn't a panic attack.

It happens again the next morning and suddenly there are five nurses in my room. Equipment is brought up from intensive care. I'm smothered under a fast-operating electric blanket. The nurses tell me that this is a sudden fever. I didn't know a fever could be so violent. I resort to an old trick which my mother taught me in my childhood. Start at four hundred, breathe deeply, and count backwards. The concentration that this requires steadies the mind. Stephen arrives at the hospital and Dr Vermeulen comes to see us.

We need to find out what the infection is, she tells me. We may be able to treat it with antibiotics, but it's possible that, in order to do that, we may have to end the pregnancy.

No, I say. No. Absolutely not.

Stephen agrees with me. There is no heroism in our words, only animal instinct. We are the lion and lioness whose cubs are threatened and who will fight to the death to defend them.

I won't let you put your own life at risk, Dr Vermeulen says.

But our baby is still alive and you've got to give her a chance.

I will be making this decision. Not you. This infection is serious enough to kill you.

I don't hear those last words and neither does Stephen. We're not even slightly discouraged because we're both absolutely sure that the hospital will be able to treat the infection.

Over the next two days, I have two more episodes of that violent shaking but then it doesn't come again. I'm definitely getting better. My arms are a mass of bandages and bruises but I don't mind because in three more days they'll move me to St Luke's and our baby will be delivered. The hospital psychologist comes to see me. I ask – If my baby dies will I be able to have a funeral?

She says that I can have whatever I want.

Even though the shaking has stopped, Dr Vermeulen is still talking about ending the pregnancy. Stephen and I protest again and she agrees to wait another twenty-four hours. That time passes and she comes to see us again, admits that the situation seems a little better. Or at least we understand her words in that way. Stephen goes home and I work out that it's three full days since the last fit of shaking. So I'm feeling pretty confident now. I'm losing clots of blood the size of my fist but this surely is a sign that the infection is clearing? As they take me down for that last scan, I have no doubt that everything will work out well and so I chat cheerily to the hospital staff and fail to notice that no one is talking to me any more.

Dr Vermeulen does the scan and I see our baby there and her heart is beating and she looks lovely. But Dr Vermeulen tells me that the waters have broken and that the pregnancy is 'condemned'. She uses this word because she's not a native speaker of English but I forgive her because it's a word which at least has the benefit of leaving me in absolutely no doubt as to what the situation is. A nurse is beside me holding my arm so tightly that it hurts.

You have had too many drugs, Dr Vermeulen tells me. They will have affected the baby – and she is just too small. She will not survive the labour.

I should question this but I don't. This is how she said it would be, no grey areas.

I'm all right, I say. I'll be OK. But I don't want our baby to suffer. She needs to die peacefully inside me. Will that be possible? Can you just leave her inside me until she's dead?

Dr Vermeulen and the nurse tell me that, of course, this is possible. But then they start to mention staff availability and timetables. And gradually I understand that they can't leave her inside me because of the infection and the risk to my health. And so they tell me that they'll induce the labour in the morning.

Initially I don't understand. Surely they'll just give me a general anaesthetic and I'll wake up when it's all over? But no. I will have to go through labour and, because of the infection, they can't give me an epidural or any other drugs except morphine. I am wheeled back up to the maternity ward and parked in a delivery room. Someone finds a mobile phone and I call Stephen. He's in the process of putting Thomas to bed and a clear picture of the two of them emerges in my mind. Standing halfway up the stairs, in the yellow light of the hall, Stephen is feeding Thomas's arms into his pyjama top. He stops to take the call.

I'm sorry but we've lost our baby.

The silence is long. At some level, I have known for some time that this would happen. But Stephen, I know, has never even considered the possibility.

What do I do? he says. I've never heard him ask that question before.

Later Stephen will tell me what happened after that call. By chance, just as he finishes talking to me, his phone rings again. It is a friend, Ben, calling for some unrelated reason. But as soon as he understands what's happened, he immediately offers to come and take Thomas. And minutes later he is at the house, gathering up Thomas's clothes for the next day, somehow making Thomas think that this is all some great adventure. Once Stephen has waved goodbye to them, he drives to the hospital and sits beside me in the delivery room.

What shall we call her? I say. I want her to have a name.

I don't know, he says. But – I like the name Laura.

I look up at him, his face floating above me in the half light of the delivery room.

That's so weird. That's the name I had imagined too.

And that's the only good moment that either of us can remember in all of that time.

It's night-time now and the nurses are already giving me the drugs which will start the labour. But I can still feel our baby moving inside me and I'm worried that she might be in distress. I try to ask one of the nurses about this.

No, she says. No. She may still be moving but she can't live.

I know she's going to die. But I don't want her to be in pain.

The nurse shows me a button I can press on the drip in my arm.

This is morphine, she says. Morphine travels across the placenta and passes from the mother's blood into the baby.

I start to press the button and I keep pressing it until I drift into sleep. Is Laura dying now? I don't know. At least she's not alone. Plenty of people are with her – Stephen, my mum, Amanda, Matthew, Rachel and Miranda. Perhaps that is what prayer is, simply recognising the significance of a person or an event. Bearing witness, saying simply – this matters. It is not death we fear, I think, only that death should prove trivial, insignificant.

The next morning I'm given more drugs. Stephen sits beside me and I wait, pressing the morphine button to ease the pain. The labour lasts for eighteen hours and three times I hear the cries of other newborn babies – that sharp, anguished cry. The cry that we're not going to hear. Around me Dr Vermeulen and the nurses are silent.

Labour. We use that word because bringing a baby into the

world is a great project, a huge undertaking. Except in this case the project has already failed.

After eight hours, I say – I can't do this any more. I can't.

But even as I speak I know that there's no point in saying this.

Later I try to say something more but when I get halfway through a sentence, I forget what I was saying. The delivery room is crowded with people. Stephen's face is so white that it's blue. I am fighting now for something more fundamental than words. *Yea though I walk through the valley of the shadow of death, I will fear no evil.* Dr Vermeulen does four blood transfusions because the bleeding doesn't stop. I'm floating away into light and silence.

Then I feel hands deep inside me and a violent wrenching. I open my eyes to see a nurse lift Laura out from between my legs and I stretch up my arms to take hold of her. After all this time, I'm excited to see her. And what do I see? Some knot of cells, some object less than human? No. What I see is someone who is more fully human than anyone I've ever seen before. This is the essence of a life, the blueprint from which the person will emerge.

She is dark red, bony, beautiful. Her soul is visible under her skin. Her face is feline, eternal. It has the serenity of an Egyptian mask. Every detail is complete – fingers, toes, eyebrows, the perfect globe of her head, marked by a mesh of veins, the fan of her tiny ribs. She's warm in my arms and surely only sleeping?

IV

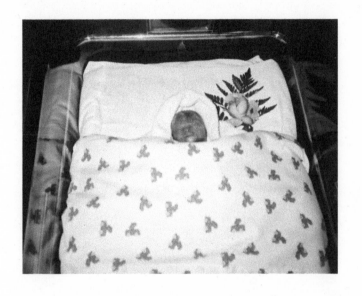

'To the world a baby, to us the world.'

Inscription on the grave
of a stillborn baby

Me-me-me, moi-moi-moi. I don't trust memoirs, never have. And I can't find the right voice. Usually I love a luscious sentence, a phrase turned with the same precision that a carpenter might use in shaping a curvaceous table leg or a bulging stair bannister. Each word cut and polished with the same care that a jeweller uses as he tends a precious stone. But when I'm teaching I say to my students – The style needs to fit the subject matter. This is Laura's story and she wanted life. It would be an insult to offer her mere literature, a crime to make the ugly beautiful.

And yet words are one of the few ways in which we can bring the dead back to life, or create a life for someone who never lived. The blossom in the Brussels gardens during that short spring, the sound of the trams, the patch of sunlight on the hospital wall – are these details a dishonest attempt to soften the sharp edges? Maybe – but they are also the world that she and I briefly occupied together. Part of what writing does is to tame horror by pinning it down into precise words. So is it such a crime for me to do that?

When I teach an anxious student, I say – Just keep writing down what you see, note the exact textures and colours, the shape of a beam of light, the warp and weft of things. Note the particular twists and turns in the grain of wood, the line of black under a fingernail, the scuffed toe of a shoe, the outline of an aerial on a roof, the geography of a cloud. Just keep recording the surfaces. The rest will take care of itself. Because it's on the surface that you find the depths.

When I wake from the general anaesthetic, they bring her to me. She's lying in a plastic hospital crib, wrapped up to her chin in a baby sheet decorated with tiny blue cars. A flower has been placed next to her head. Her skin is dark now, almost black, and she looks stiff. Her flesh is shrinking so that her skull shows through behind her face. Her bottom jaw is sagging, the lower part of her face caving in. I feel as though I should pick her up but I'm frightened. She looks so brittle she might break.

The nurses put her crib beside my bed. Evening has come again and Stephen has gone to look after Thomas and so Laura and I are alone together. For once the construction work has stopped. The sky at the window has a pink evening glow. I tell Laura about all the people in her family who would have liked to have met her. I know that soon the hospital staff will come and take her away. A nurse appears and I think that the moment has come, but she says – Is there anything you want to be buried with her?

I'm wearing my grandmother's wedding ring and I wonder if should slide that onto a ribbon and tie it around her neck. But the ring belonged to my paternal grandmother who died when I was six, and I'm not in touch with my father, so the ring is the only link I have to half of my heritage. And also I don't have a piece of ribbon. I telephone Stephen and he isn't in favour of the idea. The nurse appears and, as she wants to take Laura away, she pushes me to decide.

Once the casket is closed then it can't be reopened, she says.

Still I can't decide and so they take her away and I have given her nothing.

The hospital priest comes to visit. He's a young man with sparkling white teeth, thick black hair and a gold ring in his ear. He explains various formalities. Normally in these situations, parents need to go to the Hôtel de Ville in the Commune of Uccle and register both the birth and the death at the same time. Happily we will not have to go through all these difficulties because Laura died two days before twenty-four weeks of gestation so she doesn't need either a birth certificate or a death certificate. In fact, she doesn't have any existence in law.

I consider suggesting to the priest that he should go down to the morgue and take a look at Laura, see if he thinks that she exists. But I don't say that because he's already embarrassed and he didn't make the law, it isn't his fault.

Laura is close, I can hear her crying. It's three days since she died but her voice is everywhere, screaming for me. I stand up and my head spins, my stomach lurches. I steady myself against the hospital bed. My feet shuffle as I take hold of the drip stand and push it towards the door. I struggle to get out of the room and then wander down the dipping and swaying corridor, under the harsh white lights, looking for Laura. I am aware that there's something theatrical in this. Something of the Victorian lunatic asylum, the straitjacket, the scold's bridle. I know that she is dead but I want to shock, I want to rave and froth at the mouth.

A nurse appears and asks me what I'm doing. I tell her that I'm looking for my baby, that I can hear her crying. More nurses appear, watching me uncertainly. I'm guided back to my room and put to bed. A young woman doctor comes, not someone I've met before. She sits down by the bed, tells me that she has recently lost her mother. Of course you feel your baby close to you, she says. That's because she is.

After the doctor has gone, the nurses disconnect the drip from my arm because I'm meant to be going home. But I don't want to leave the hospital because, while I'm here, I'm obviously ill. Outside the hospital I'll be expected to continue with my life. I'll need to put the washing machine on, hang clothes on the line, load the dishwasher, write my novel, wipe Thomas's nose. I can't do those things. But Stephen is coming to pick me up in an hour so I need to get to the bathroom, wash and clean my teeth, pack up my belongings.

I can't find the strength. I stare around me, looking at all the details of the room – the television screen, books, photographs, and that sock, that mysterious pink sock with the blue flower stitched onto the cuff – all things which were here when Laura was alive. Life boils itself down to a simple choice. Either I have to go and clean my teeth or I'm going to finish up in the psychiatric ward of the hospital. It's Laura who provides me with the strength to get to the bathroom. She cannot have died in order for me to finish up mad. There must be some other purpose to all of this.

When Stephen arrives he finishes packing up the room and takes everything down to the car. Then he comes back to help me. We discuss the pink sock that still lies on the table under the television. Stephen thinks we should leave it but I can't be parted from it. I need to find the child who owns it, I must do that.

As we emerge into the corridor, a scuffle is taking place around the lifts. Soon it becomes apparent that a tactful nurse is trying to clear the corridor of mothers, babies and smiling relatives before we pass by. But her efforts are thwarted and Stephen I are squeezed into the lift with the families who have live babies. Balloons bob in our faces and smiling relatives grip crackling-cellophane flowers, babygrows, teddy bears. Stephen and I stare at the floor. He's holding a packet that contains a blurred photograph of Laura.

I get home to find that some maternity clothes that I ordered have arrived. The package contains a cheery note wishing me well for the rest of my pregnancy. I finish up wearing the clothes as I can't fit into any others. I'm so weak that I can barely walk but I go out to get my hair cut. The hairdresser asks when the baby is due. On the way there, I meet a woman whom I know well. The look of terror on her face confirms that she knows what has happened but she talks about nothing, hurries on. Hidden shallows. I am about to discover that they are everywhere.

I still have the rash. My breasts hurt, my feet are swollen. I have anaemia and I'm still bleeding. Usually after a pregnancy you hardly notice these things because you're so in love with your baby. Flowers and cards arrive but no one speaks to us. The silence moves through my body, freezing my muscles and bones, one by one. I am trapped in a besieged city, sending out endless distress signals, but no one can hear.

The world of Dead Babies is a silent and shuttered place. You do not know it exists until you find yourself there. I read on the internet that in the UK seventeen babies are stillborn every day. What has happened to us isn't rare, extraordinary. So then why have I never known about it? Because stillbirths are taboo – and the whole point about a taboo is that you don't know it's there until you step right into the middle of it.

Late at night, unable to sleep, that question runs riot in my head. Why didn't I know that this could happen? I go downstairs, sit at the computer in Stephen's study and open the website of Sands, the Stillbirth and Neonatal Death Charity. I find my way into the forum – surely the bleakest acre of cyberspace. There they are, the tiny babies – shown in blurred photographs – with their cradles, babygrows, white cotton hats and teddy bears. All of them perfect, all of them dead. These babies are surrounded by tiny memorials – pictures of storks, hearts and flowers. Ticker tapes which measure the days. *Six months and fifteen days since our Angel Liam got his wings.* A link to click so you can light an online candle. *Two months and seven days until our Angel Sarah's first birthday.* Poems and messages. *Most people only dream of angels, we held one in our arms.* To me, this all seems rather weird and sentimental.

I click onto the section of personal stories. A significant number of them are about women who have had a perfectly normal full-term pregnancy and then also have a normal, easy labour – but then the baby never breathes and no one is ever able to tell them why.

I was unaware that this still happened. Surely there must be a medical explanation? The whole thing seems Victorian, archaic. It's a level of tragedy which shouldn't exist in a modern society – and yet it does. I'm not someone who uses the internet much but I sign up for the discussion forum and enter an unending world of loss, hundreds of stories, hundreds of comments, hundreds of photographs, hundreds of Dead Babies.

Why didn't I know that this was here? The information is overwhelming – and insulting. I note down the help line number but then I can't look any more. I don't want to read about anyone else's loss. I want my grief to be bigger and better than any other grief. I want Laura to be the only baby who has ever died. She mustn't be lost among that great cyber army of the dead with their little white hats and ghostly eyes, their blurred faces and grey skin. I shut the computer down and head back upstairs, lie in bed, sleepless.

We go back to the hospital to get the results of the autopsy. I sit on a bench sandwiched between a heavily pregnant woman and another who is breastfeeding. When Dr Vermeulen does a scan neither Stephen nor I look at the screen. The autopsy reveals what we always knew. There was nothing the matter with Laura. She was a perfectly healthy little girl.

So how come she's dead?

The support system on which she depended – the placenta – gradually failed. It happens sometimes. We don't know why.

Dr Vermeulen shakes her head, comments that I'm lucky to have survived.

And now, she says. About the next pregnancy. You are thirty-eight years old. I know, you were waiting three years for the one you've just lost. You have no time to waste.

I feel anger swamp me. Her words blur and twist. I have a baby and I don't want another. I watch her lips but hear no sounds. Stephen is asking whether a detached placenta is a condition that can recur. And although I'm not listening, I realise that no decisive reassurance has been offered. Yes, perhaps, one cannot say. Certainly there are risks. As with everything else the risk increases as you get older.

I leave the room in a blazing rage. Who is this other baby who thinks to take Laura's place?

As we leave the hospital, Stephen has to go to the administration department to fill out a form so I head back to the car on my own. As I step into the lift which will take me down to the car park, I realise that, among the crowds around me, there is a woman with a baby in a Maxi-Cosi. I try to push my way out again but I'm too late. The doors have closed, the lift is dropping downwards. I turn my head away, breathe deeply, clench my fists.

The baby starts to cry – first a grizzling snuffle but then a full volume wail which burns into my flesh, my bones, like acid. I press my head against the wall of the lift, pray that soon we'll reach our destination. The baby continues to wail and bile rises in my throat. When the lift finally bumps to a stop, I stagger out and my knees buckle. So I sink down against the wall and hide my face in my hands.

Stephen and I decide we'll take Laura back to England so she can be buried in the Church of the Good Shepherd at The Hook – which is the village in Worcestershire where my mum lives. That church is only a few hundred yards down the road from Mum's farm and we often walk the dogs there in the evening. Stephen and I were married in that church, and Thomas was christened there. The date is set for three days after our fourth wedding anniversary. A for Anderlecht, B for Boitsfort, C for Châtelain, D for Death.

As Laura does not exist in law, then surely it should be easy enough to take her home? But no – undertakers don't deal with a body if there isn't a death certificate, the airlines won't let us fly, customs can't confirm that we'll be able to enter the UK. The British Embassy don't want to know, even though we know many of the people there. Stephen would normally be able to cut his way through all this easily but he's lost his powers of decision-making. He panics and fumbles his way through minor administrative tasks. I find him one night glued to the computer screen, trying yet again to find a way to get her home.

Listen, I say. Stop worrying. We're going to get her home somehow. If we have to hide her in the boot of the car and drive through the ferry ports then we'll do that. The chance that we'll be searched is more or less nil.

And so that's what we plan to do. But before Stephen has booked the ferry, a mysterious phone call comes from Eurostar offering to transport us back to the UK. And so Stephen makes a booking and we go to the hospital to get the coffin. We need to find the morgue but there are no signs. At the reception desk they look shocked when I ask, as though I have said something offensive. Finally we find the tiny, unmarked slip road that leads down to the basement which houses the morgue.

We are led into a bare room and see the coffin on a table. It's not much more than eighteen inches long and made of shiny pine, the lid held in place by four ornate brass knobs. Usually I hate shiny pine but I'm pleased by the coffin. It looks just right. A white flower is placed on the top of it. The hospital priest helps us put the coffin in the boot of the car. Then he watches us drive up the slip road and across the car park, standing silently at the door of the morgue until we're out of sight. I think he knows how long our journey will be.

For one night Laura is at home with us and I want the house to be clean and white and spacious, so that she can occupy it in peace. But everything is such chaos that we struggle to find a place to put her. Finally Stephen clears the end of the dining room table while I find a baby blanket of bright crocheted squares to put under her. That white flower still lies on the lid of the coffin although it's beginning to look withered now. I wish that we could just keep her here forever but, as always, there is no time.

Tomorrow we have to get the Eurostar and the packing isn't done yet. And I'm meant to be going to a meeting of my Writers' Group. Should I go or not? Decisions like that seem very unimportant now. In fact, all decisions have become irrelevant. Nothing will change the reality of what has happened. Finally I decide not to go out and instead I sit by the coffin, writing in my diary, describing again and again the exact details of the coffin, the blanket, the white flower. Holding her here, keeping her with us. She's so close that I could just gather her into my arms.

The next morning we put Laura's coffin into a holdall, bundle Thomas into his pushchair and set out for the Gare du Midi. Eurostar take us through the VIP lounge and a lovely man apologises twenty times because they have to put the coffin through the security scan. On the train, we have a whole carriage to ourselves. I think it was the priest at the hospital who organised this. We leave the train at Ashford so that we can pick up a hire car. Stephen and Thomas carry the holdall through the station, each holding one handle. Carrying her coffin in a holdall seems both disrespectful and absolutely right. Is it so very different from the carrycot we would have used if she had lived?

We head for my mother's farm, which lies at the foot of the Malvern Hills, above the town of Upton upon Severn. As we near the farm, Thomas wants us to do a countdown, as we usually do. Thirty, twenty-nine, twenty-eight. We take the shaded road out of Upton upon Severn, and head up past Clive's Fruit Farm and over the old railway bridge. Nineteen, eighteen, seventeen. The mellow red brick of the semi-derelict farmhouse and the Dutch barn are visible up ahead. Five, four, three. My mother is waiting at the gate. She is suddenly old. Two, one. Thomas cheers.

That evening I go down with flu. I worry that the infection from the hospital has started again. It hasn't but still I'm shivering and sit by the fire wrapped in a duvet. The rash returns and at night I lie awake, feverish and itching. I worry that I might not be able to get out of bed for the funeral. At least the bleeding has finally stopped and that should be a relief. But strangely I mourn for it. I was bleeding for Laura, I'd have bled every drop in my body if it could have been enough.

What I want to do is go to the sea – the farm isn't near the sea but it's only one and a half hours down the M5 to Weston-super-Mare. If only I could get there, I would feel better. I dream of Ostend, Brighton, that massive stone house near Aberdovey and the deserted station. What made us turn away and run for home? Who inhabited that place? And what, if anything, does that person, that force, have to do with Laura's death?

Next morning, when the house is empty, I go down to the sitting room to look at Laura's coffin. We have placed her next to the sideboard on a table covered with a white cloth. At her feet are a cluster of flowers sent by neighbours. I like having Laura at the farm with us, I like her neat little coffin and I dread the moment when she will have to leave. I have the usual sense of a moment squandered, insufficiently appreciated, insufficiently lived. Should I not have sat by the coffin all day and all night? That is what they would have done in the old days.

Instead I pick the coffin up, finding it surprisingly heavy, and carry it upstairs to the bedroom. I lay it down next to me, amidst the piles of eiderdowns and blankets. The curtains at the window are half open and I lie there staring out at the fat green leaves on the oak tree that stands on the back drive. A strong wind blows and they dance and twist, their colours changing in the shifting light.

A letter has arrived from my father and lies on the bedside table. I decide that the moment has come to open it, take some deep breaths. I wrote to him a week ago to tell him of Laura's death because, although he refuses to speak to me, I felt he had a right to know. Now I read his response. As always I'm struck by his prose – precise, elegant, each cadence perfectly placed. Flawless words used as a means of saying nothing. Apparently he is able to imagine that the situation must be upsetting. I had expected no more and I put the letter aside and drift into sleep.

I wake to hear Thomas on the creaking stairs. He has come back from a country fair that he has been to with my mum. He's been riding on quad bikes and playing minigolf. He climbs up onto the bed to tell me about it and lines his toy animals up on the coffin. A plastic cow, a collie dog, a pig and two chickens. This is my baby sister, he says proudly, patting the lid of the coffin. I don't mind if she plays with my animals. She can play with them any time.

My mum comes and takes him back downstairs. The house is empty once again and I drift back into sleep, with Laura still lying next to me. When I wake, the light has changed and the day is waning. I hear careful footsteps on the creaking stairs and the handle of the bedroom door turns. Our friend Matthew has arrived from Hay-on-Wye. He enters the room and sees me under the duvet with the coffin next to me. He comes over to kiss me and then stands back.

Sorry, I say, indicating the coffin. You must think I've gone a bit cranky?

No, he says. No. In fact, seeing you like that makes me know you'll be all right sometime.

Later I get up and walk with my mum down the fields, still wearing a wool dressing gown over two jumpers. As we walk, we look over to the Malvern Hills, which rise to the left of us. This farm used to belong to my mother's friend, Verity, who left it to our family in her will, and so I have known the land here for many years. But the hills never cease to surprise, appearing from nowhere, jutting steeply upwards, a knife-edge ridge in the earth – dark and high – blocking out the sun. As a child, I found them sinister and unwelcoming but over the years I've grown used to their brooding presence.

Mum and I don't talk much. As always, she has puppies in the fallen-down stables and foals out in the rutted, dock-leaf-scattered fields. And I remember now how, as a child, we often stayed up late into the night bottle-feeding orphaned lambs, or dripping milk into fragile puppies with a tiny dropper, and how sometimes, despite all our efforts, we found a puppy or a lamb stiff and cold in the morning, smelling of death. And no one could tell us why.

Do you remember? I say to my mother. That litter of puppies. Labradors. They belonged to Mr Smith on the farm next door. And we went over to see them. Do you remember? And then the next day we heard that they were all dead because the bitch had slept on them and suffocated them all.

Yes, my mother does remember.

And the foals, she says. You've seen it, haven't you? More than once?

I know what she's talking about: those times when a foal is expected and Mum is out in the fields late at night, checking the mare, especially if it's a fine night, as foals are never born in the rain. But then, early in the morning, I hear her calling up to me from the yard, her voice strangled by tears, and I leap up and pull on my clothes, hurry down the field and the foal is there – dead, the dew settled on its soft baby fur.

You know, my mother says. People who don't have much experience of these things talk endlessly about Mother Nature and the miracles of the natural world. But Darwin didn't say that. Instead he said that natural processes are largely characterised by appallingly high levels of waste.

The funeral takes place on a June day, which is neither hot nor cold, with a sky as blank as a sheet of paper. Stephen and I pick up the coffin and carry it down the deserted country lane to the Church of the Good Shepherd. I walked this same road to the church four years ago on our wedding day. We need a stand to put the coffin on and so Matthew carries a card table from the sitting room and brings with it a white cloth. Our writer friend Adam, from Brussels, has come to the funeral despite his illness, the distance, the difficulties of leaving Miranda with three small children.

The church looks very fine with its altar cloth of pale green and gold. Matthew places the table up near the choir stalls and my mother organises the white cloth so that the lace edge of it hangs straight around the table. Then she brings the four white roses from the garden in a jam jar and puts them at the foot of the coffin. I don't think that four garden roses in a jam jar have ever looked so radiant.

At the last minute it seems that the vicar expects me to read from the Bible. I can't do it so I pass the Bible to Matthew and he does it instead. *Suffer the little children and forbid them not to come unto me, for of such is the kingdom of heaven ... And whoever receives a little child in my name receives me.* The service finishes with the Celtic Blessing. *And until we meet again, may God keep you safe in the hollow of His hand.*

Thomas is silent throughout, standing with Stephen's mother, watching. At the end of the service, we take Laura outside and lay her down in the newly cut earth. It feels just like tucking her up in her cot, making her comfortable for the night. On her gravestone are the words – *Before I formed you in the womb, I knew you. Jeremiah 1:5.* I realise that, for everyone else, this is finished now. For us, it's never going to end.

After the funeral, we all walk back to the farm and sit in the kitchen, drinking tea, then whisky. A neighbour has made cakes but no one feels like eating them. I sit at the kitchen table, blank and drained. A friend of my mother's says – You know those new speakers you were talking about. The portable ones. My daughter-in-law has just got them and she says they work really well.

I stare at her, bemused, and she sidles away, realising that she has hit the wrong note. But I'm always grateful to that friend because, over all the years that have passed since that day, whenever I think of that particular moment, I laugh. Catastrophe and comedy walk hand in hand.

V

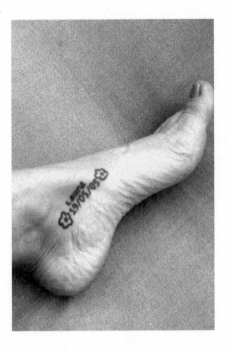

I know your sorrow and I know for the likes of us there is no ease for the heart to be had from words of reason and that in the very assurance of sorrow fading there is more sorrow. So I offer you only my deeply affectionate and compassionate thoughts and wish for you only that the strange thing may never fail you, whatever it is, that gives us the strength to live on and on with our wounds.

Samuel Beckett

I don't trust memoirs, never have. They do not allow the case for the defence to be heard. And although the memoir writer may set out to portray events accurately, the endeavour always fails because, when we write about the past, we organise it. We make it like a novel – with a beginning, a middle, an end, a chain of cause and effect, a degree of resolution. Although I work with that process all day, I distrust it when applied to the scattered realities of daily life. Wordsworth famously described poetry as strong emotion recollected in tranquillity. But I want to write the emotions without the tranquillity, without the help or hindrance of hindsight. I don't want resolution. I never want to look back and say – *I can see now that it was all for the best.*

Now, in my non-existent life, in this Gloucestershire world of football boots and dawn drives across Rodborough Common, now – in this long period of waiting – I send the barrister the last of the information which she needs for the High Court hearing. So I can now put the cardboard box away. The chronology has been established – more or less – although I never did find that missing year. And yet I keep writing, writing for you, Laura. Using words to raise the dead.

Tell me, my dear, how does one describe absence?

Because absence is all you are.

Perhaps it's like making a stencil, a craft project that you and I might have worked on together, on a winter's afternoon at Mount Vernon, after a walk on Rodborough Common, with the wood-burning stove alight in the playroom, sitting by the bay window, with the evening advancing across the valley, the lights of Stroud appearing far below.

Take a piece of thin card, my love, and a pair of scissors with tips as sharp as needles. Then start to cut a shape. Work slowly, in good light. Turn the card, not the scissors, as you work. Find the shape as you cut, feel it growing through the tips of your fingers. Cut and snip and cut. Do not allow your hands to shake or jerk.

When you are finished, tape the card to a pale wall. Dip a blunt-ended brush into the paint, then wipe most of the colour away. Dab with the brush against the wall, slowly filling the hole in the card. Allow the paint to dry thoroughly, peel back the card and a shape will appear on the wall – blurred perhaps and faint, but still a definite shape.

Could this work, my love? If I measure your absence with words, snip and cut and turn, then will some shadow of your presence appear on the wall? We both of us know that it will not be so. You are not here, you never were.

Grief is a disastrous subject for a book. It is slippery, episodic, repetitive. It lacks shape, or landmarks, clearly defined paths. It is a journey leading nowhere, a quest to solve the one problem that can never have a solution. Before Laura died, I thought grief might contain some element of glamour. Perhaps a woman sitting on a sofa, weeping elegantly, surrounded by caring friends bringing wisdom and home-made lasagne?

But the reality bears no resemblance to that cosy fantasy. I read about grief on various websites. They make it sound like a third form geography project – first you go through denial and isolation, then anger, bargaining, depression. My own experience defies such categories. I can begin a sentence in denial and end it in anger, having made a bargain with God en route.

After the funeral, back in Brussels the merry-go-round days jangle on. My publishers are demanding my long overdue novel so I try to write but can't. I need movement, constant movement. So I pull my bike out of the garage, set off down the Chaussée d'Ixelles towards the centre of the city, pedalling hard, weaving in and out of the racing and squealing traffic – to the Grand Place and then out to the canals, back via the Rue de la Loi, the Parc du Cinquantenaire, Les Etangs d'Ixelles.

Most people dismiss the city of Brussels before they've taken the trouble to know it. It is seen as the posting you are given if you've missed out on Paris or New York. But Stephen and I have always loved Brussels, it is our home, and now its physical details are all that can save me. Cycle, just keep cycling. And when exhaustion finally overwhelms you, sit down in a café and write, describe the streets around you. Do that for long enough and you will be overwhelmed by the sheer wonder that any of this exists at all. And that feeling will obliterate all others.

I cycle out through St Gilles, to the Gare du Midi and beyond to Anderlecht and Molenbeek St Jean. Then St Josse, the Basilique. The worst thing that could possibly happen has already happened and I'm still alive. The city dashes past me in swirls of brown and red. The trees raise their branches in shock, the mouths of tunnels gape, the tramlines glitter like traps. The brakes of the trams shriek. The Art Nouveau window frames are twisted up, the tall houses bend in on me – but still I do not stop. I am euphorically, indecently happy. I hear Laura's voice – *You better live because I cannot.*

In the evenings, after cooking the supper and getting Thomas off to bed, I save the world. Join Greenpeace, Friends of the

Earth, read books about eradicating World Poverty, install low energy light bulbs throughout the house, position bricks in the loo cisterns to save water. I am restless, powerful, invincible. Because Laura has died, we have to become better people. If we don't, then her short life had no meaning. Laura has bequeathed me her courage and I've become the brave person I always wanted to be. Go here, there, buy the right skirt, get the right haircut, see this person, fix this, fix that. Outwit death for one more day.

Later – much later – I find myself talking to a vicar about those weeks after Laura's funeral. And, strangely, I tell this man, whom I don't know, something which I've never admitted to anyone else. Which is that for weeks after her death, I found myself hot with the need for sex, like a dog on heat, like a man who fucks a prostitute in an alleyway. I tell the vicar this because I felt guilty. A stillbirth may be a traumatic shock to the hormonal system but is that really an adequate excuse?

The vicar is both unembarrassed by my confession, and unsurprised. Apparently in his profession it's well known that at funerals it's best not to open doors because you never know what you might find behind them. Couples copulating on the couch, fiddling against the freezer, groping in the garden shed, bonking in the basement.

The vicar tells me that the overwhelming desire to have sex that sometimes comes over people at funerals has to do with the need to celebrate life in the face of death. Because the two are inextricably linked. Because the death of one person reaffirms the life of another.

You're doing pretty well at this Dead Baby business, I tell myself. I read some of the more hysterical entries on the Sands website – women who are suicidal, who simply can't find a way to get through the day – and congratulate myself on not making too much fuss. I decide on a basic mantra and repeat it again and again – *We're all doing fine. This isn't Zimbabwe or the Horn of Africa.*

But what I have failed to understand – such mercy in ignorance – is that the process of grief hasn't even started yet. I am still in shock – kindly protective shock. People in shock get divorced, emigrate, resign from their job, refuse to speak to their family and friends but they feel nothing except a buzzing, listless energy. I know now that shock is a gift and should be welcomed. It catapults you into some alternative universe that is unpredictable and dangerous but better than the pain from which it is designed to protect you.

I go to the Quaker Meeting House and my news is received there in silence – a profound, generous, silence. I know this response speaks of the fact that the Friends consider my loss to be too great to be encompassed by mere words and I am grateful. But still I want answers so I borrow books from the Meeting House library, read late into sleepless nights.

My mind goes back again to that morning on the coast in Wales. I've always envied atheists. What a luxury to simply not believe in God. Regrettably I have always experienced God – or some similar force – so powerfully that the question of belief is rendered irrelevant. And I've always wanted – longed – to understand more about that force but now my need has become urgent. Whether God exists or not, I have business to settle with Him.

All the books about Buddhism, meditation and prayer are

interesting but they none of them provide the answers I am seeking. They are too big, too abstract, too wandering. I may not be able to write my novel any more but still I need narrative, a story to steady my mind. It doesn't need to be original or interesting. In fact, any level of cliché is acceptable as long as the story is sufficiently small and concrete to carry me through the day.

And so this is what I tell myself: Stephen and I are embarking on a long process of getting to know Laura. We will not organise a first birthday party for her, we will not see her take her first step. We will not wave to her as she sets off for her first day at school. We will not attend her wedding or hold her child in our arms. And all down the long years we will be haunted by those events that do not happen.

And yet at some other level we are going to get to know her. That knowing will not consist of physical things – nappies, sleepless nights, Cornish holidays, schoolbooks or parent–teacher evenings. Instead it will be a knowing of the mind, of the spirit. Gradually we will understand why Laura became part of our lives. She came to offer us something, or reveal something. But our understanding of this will not come quickly. We must wait patiently on the process. It may take months, or even years. Perhaps a lifetime. At present, all that is required is the faith to know that this will happen. On the good days – taking the train out to the coast, walking along the seafront at Ostend or De Haan – I am sure of this.

On the bad days, while Thomas is at nursery, I spend long hours reading the stories on the Sands website. One day I find an account written by a woman whose baby was born alive at twenty-two weeks. Then I find more of the same. None of the tiny babies in these stories lived for more than a few hours –

but they were born alive. Their mothers give the times with scalpel precision.

James alive for fourteen minutes.

Sasha alive for thirty-seven minutes.

Twins. Jordan one hour, twenty-two minutes. Ben one hour, forty minutes.

But we were told that Laura, delivered at twenty-four weeks, couldn't possibly be born alive. That wasn't true. I lay my head down on the desk beside the computer and swallow back a mouthful of bile. Could the hospital have saved Laura? The nausea I feel is not so much the shock of revelation but the bitter realisation that I've been avoiding this question.

And can do so no longer.

Friends have told us that we should sue the hospital for medical negligence but Stephen and I have ignored them. We agree that these people aren't really talking about our story. Instead they are suffering from that modern disease – an inability to accept that sometimes bad things happen and no one is at fault. To me, it's always been clear that Laura's death was just bad luck.

But now I begin to wonder. Could the hospital have done more?

We never insisted, questioned. And that now is the real question – why did we not fight for her? I don't know. Somehow I just accepted that she had to die. Now I read the words of those other mothers. They say – I don't care how badly disabled my baby would have been, I just want my baby. I just want my baby, no matter what.

But the bitter truth is that I don't feel like that. During those tortured days in the hospital, I was haunted by the image of a tiny baby, full of tubes and wires, suffering, irreparably damaged. Haunted by the thought of what that would have done to her, to Thomas, to me, to all of our family.

I prefer Laura as she is – perfect and dead, at peace.

I'm not a saint, I'm not even an averagely good person.

The situation can't now be changed. But still I could have had twenty minutes, or half an hour. I could have felt her heart beat, maybe even seen her eyes looking at me. I could have had a photograph of a live baby. So why didn't I?

I ask Stephen this question.

You know that near the end of the labour there was that great big wrenching? I say. I felt it inside me. I reckon Dr Vermeulen killed Laura because she didn't want her to come out alive. Do you think that could be right?

I look at Stephen and I realise that I've gone too far, much too far. He is doing his best to live with my constant questioning, my determination to investigate and examine. But this is too much and I should have known it.

It's too much for me as well. But still I consider going back to the hospital to talk to Dr Vermeulen, not to blame or accuse, only to understand. But I can't face going. Finally I don't blame Dr Vermeulen. Instead I'm grateful to her. She took a decision for us that we could never have taken ourselves. She didn't want us to be left with guilt as well as grief. But still I mourn for that fifteen minutes we could have had.

Every day Stephen and I walk through a minefield. Anything might cause the world to break apart: a little girl's dress in a shop window, a mother with a pushchair, a picture of a sick or starving child, a random comment about how tiring it is to look after a baby. The mines go off all the time, taking an arm or a leg with them, ripping flesh off the bone.

But we have to keep on walking, keep on inhabiting the world of living children and babies. We have no choice, we have a three-year-old son. Every woman we know is either pregnant or has a newborn baby. Our social life consists of children's parties and outings to the park. Babies are every-where. All I can do is walk past them with my teeth gritted and try not to see. We have to do this for Thomas. Stephen and I have talked about this and we are agreed – he is not going to pay for his sister's death.

He asks questions all the time.

Mummy, do people who are dead ever come alive again? Mummy, how can our baby grow if she's in a box in the ground? Mummy, why was she born too early? Mummy, can we go out to the shops and buy a new baby at the weekend? Mummy, don't be sad because you're making me sad as well. And mainly – I don't understand why she died.

I try to respond although I don't have any answers. Some-times he goes on and on and won't be distracted. Will I die soon? Will you die? Why did she die? Why? Where is she? Where? And I just want to say – Will you shut up? But he has his process of grief to go through and it is my job to help him. And so I keep on answering.

Mummy, Mummy, can I ask you a question?

Yes, darling. Are you worrying about Laura again?

No. I just want to know – do stick insects get car sick?

Where is Laura? Where? His question is my question. Is she wearing one pink sock with a tiny blue flower stitched onto the cuff? Sometimes when I'm sitting at the computer, trying to write, a bubble pops up containing a message. *Sarah wants to chat with you. Kelly wants to chat with you.* Then one day – inevitably – *Laura wants to chat with you.*

So she's there. I stop myself from clicking on the message, switch the computer off, spend the rest of the afternoon riding my bike, too fast, through the lethal Brussels traffic. That evening, when Stephen comes home, I want to tell him that I've had a message from Laura but I'll only upset him. But still I can't stop myself.

I wait until he's gone out again and type her full name – Laura Catherine Kinsella – into the search engine. She's close, so close and soon I'm going to find her. Her name comes up immediately. Laura Catherine Kinsella, deceased. With urgent, stumbling fingers I click on the link. Information about how to research and create a family tree. I scroll down and she's there. Laura Catherine Kinsella. Deceased 1813, aged six years, in Homestead, a rural area of Ontario.

She was the youngest of three children. Her mother went to a neighbour's house to get some milk, leaving the children at home. While she was out, Laura played too close to the fire and her dress caught alight. The two older children got out alive but the mother returned to find Laura and the house gone.

I scroll down further, click on other links, try the search engine again. Where is the rest of the story? What happened afterwards? Where did the family go? But there is nothing more, just that fragment. But still I see it all. The forests and the winding road, the mean wooden houses in the bottom of the valley. The sky above, white and clear, as deep as the ocean. And inside the wooden house, Laura is there. She has long brown hair, yearning eyes. Her older siblings tell her to be careful, not to go near the fire.

But she's spinning and twisting, round and round, lost inside her own head, dreaming of the future, going to the city. And as she turns her dress swirls outwards, and a wind in the chimney flares the fire. And the dress catches. And within seconds, she has gone. A bright dazzle of flame. A scream silenced. Her mouth open, her hands stretched out as the flames engulf her, dash up towards the ceiling. Catching curtains, beams, the wood of the mantelpiece.

And there's her mother, running across the road, through the still white air, her arms waving. But she is too late. And then. And then. I don't know, I can't know. But the image of Laura Catherine Kinsella, dress alight, arms stretched up, dazzling, is trapped inside my head and buzzes there for days. Forever. At least she had six years, a dress, dreams. A view of the forests and the infinite white sky. I'm running home, Laura, running across the road as fast as I can. Running to pull you out of the burning house. Wait for me please.

Brussels is closing down. Our friends Adam and Miranda are leaving permanently to live in Bordeaux. As we see them several times a week, this leaving cuts a deep wound. We never manage to say a proper goodbye. The city has an end of term feel, an atmosphere both mournful and expectant. The streets become empty and silent, shutters are pulled down. Stephen and I plant a rose bush in the garden in memory of Laura. I take the train out to the coast, walk, write my novel, read.

Finally, the day comes when we too are leaving. We load the Peugeot 106 and set off for Calais. Thomas and I are going to spend August at the farm with my mum. At the end of the long journey, Thomas counts down as we near the farm. Five, four, three. Mum is at the gate waving. Two. One. Behind her the jumble of red-brick farm buildings, the dock-leaf fields and sagging gates.

Often during those long August Worcestershire nights, I am unable to sleep and wander down to the morning room where endless pungent dogs snooze on sofas. I open the windows, hear the rustling sounds of the night-time farmyard – horses munching, a light wind creaking through the timbers of the barn. In the distance the black wall of the Malvern Hills. Then I shift a dog from the sofa, put the television on, allow my eyes to follow Open University science programmes.

One night I drift into sleep but then wake again, shift on the sofa. The Open University has gone and the camera is fixed on a man called John who is telling his story. He was the victim of a serious assault and later had a nervous breakdown. Something about the way he speaks sets an alarm bell ringing. I sit up, watch, listen.

John explains that the attack happened in broad daylight on a country road that is reasonably busy. He was driving home from work when another car came up behind him, pulled parallel with him, pushed him into the verge. Then a man jumped out, pulled him out of his car, and beat him savagely, breaking his arm and several ribs, smashing his face to a pulp.

John lay on the side of the road, bleeding badly, for about twenty minutes. During that time many cars drove past but they didn't stop. John, stuttering and twisting his hands, his face occasionally crumpling up as the muscles go into spasm, explains that it wasn't the attack that caused his breakdown. He's always known that it was the work of a random lunatic and so attaches no wider significance to it.

But it was the cars that drove past which broke him. They changed his view of the world. He thought he was living in a caring society and found out he wasn't. The interview ends, John disappears back into his own life. But for hours afterwards, I lie cramped on the sofa, in the darkness, wide awake. I've turned the television off but still I stare at the black screen. I'm thinking of the cars passing and the man called John lying bleeding by the side of the road. And he's calling out to the cars and waving his fractured arm. Waving and waving but the cars don't stop.

VI

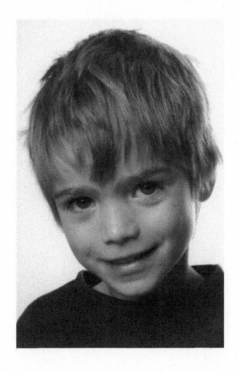

If love could have saved you,
you would have lived forever.

Anonymous / Traditional

What next? Here my pen falters. Laura, I can write your death, your funeral, those first few months of euphoric shock. I can write all that in the present tense. Pain as it is lived, without the tranquilliser of hindsight. But now I come to the rage – and I stop. How I wish I could un-know the oceans, the universes of rage which grief can unleash. A rage like a whirlwind. Capricious and divisive. A rage which attaches itself to anything and anybody. A petty, self-pitying rage that waits for someone to make a tactless comment and then nurses a violent anger against them for days, months, years. A rage which lacks any splendour, any generosity, any humour.

Even now, after seven years, I don't want to ease the cork on the bottle. The page will burn up under my pen, the globe will creak on its axis, even the stars will hide their light. There are thoughts so toxic that they must be buried deep, far out at sea, like nuclear waste. Or put down a mineshaft, covered with layer upon layer of concrete.

I grasp the steadying handrail of the rational mind. My rage, the rage of all those bereaved mothers on the Sands website. What is at the root of it? Perhaps all that happened to me is that I had an encounter with reality. But why was I so un-prepared? After all, I had already experienced difficult losses before.

I think the answer is that I accepted the world as it was publicised to me. Most of us do, even though we know we shouldn't. It's hard to avoid soaking up the images of happiness that surround us. All stories have happy endings. Adversity is overcome, conflict resolved.

And it isn't only the media who create this unreal world.

My generation of middle-class children were protected from things which were difficult. Adults whispered about tragedy but we had no experience of it. I do not particularly blame my parents for this. They accepted the received wisdom of their time.

But then the problem is that when the world finally reveals itself to be extraordinarily cruel – as it will do for nearly everyone at some time – we have no resources with which to cope. We realise that we have been living in a world of distorted mirror images and are left confused, deceived, rudderless. We stand amazed at the size of the lie and the confidence with which it has been propagated.

As individuals and as a society, we have lost the vocabulary to talk about the dark things, to tell the stories that don't have a happy ending. Which is all very well, until you find yourself in a place where you need to tell those stories. And then you will stammer and stutter, find yourself rapidly silenced. And so the rage starts, rage against silence, denial, the militant insistence that nothing has really happened.

We are all of us in denial about death. Get the dead under the sod and move on as quickly as possible. That doesn't help anyone who is bereaved, but for the parents of a stillborn baby the situation is much worse, largely because so few people have seen what has been lost. The parents of that baby feel all the emotions that every parent feels – pride, amazement and that dizzying sense that this tiny person is now the axis on which the world spins. Love so strong that it could knock you from your feet. And they continue to feel all these things long, long after the baby is buried.

But to everyone else the baby isn't real at all, never existed. They may have heard that a baby was expected. Then they hear that the baby has died. So there was no baby. And so a massive chasm exists between what the parents are seeing and feeling and what the world around them is seeing. And contained within the depth and width of this chasm is the trauma of the stillbirth.

During that Brussels autumn, I put the washing machine on, hang clothes on the line, load the dishwasher, write a short story, wipe Thomas's nose. But increasingly I am losing the battle for normality. Strangely it is my hands which are most affected. I am unable to thread a needle, tie my bootlaces or even write my name clearly. My neck and shoulders have seized up, I find it difficult to breathe. I hear through a wad of cotton wool, my eyes peer through frosted glass. I no longer write anything down in my notebooks because I no longer see.

Every month my period is late – sometimes as much as two weeks late – and I think that I'm pregnant but then it turns out that I'm not. I don't know whether to be pleased or sad but I don't like the not knowing, the waiting. I get out the scarf that I started to knit in the hospital. Because the needles are thick as pencils, I can just about handle them, if I concentrate. The rhythm of the needles is comforting. The scarf grows to two feet, then four. It is wide, thick and warm. Six feet, seven, eight. I am looking forward to wearing it, now that winter is coming on.

Stephen and I speak less and less. He's angry with me because I don't want to go anywhere, because I hate everyone we know. I don't understand why he doesn't want to talk. He is in as much pain as I am but he wants to carry on with normal life whereas I do not. I refuse to answer e-mails or phone calls. I don't speak to people when I meet them, or say something bitter or inappropriate. More and more friends are going. They are condemned without trial. They said the wrong thing or failed to say anything at all. I am gradually alienating everyone we know and feeling a warped sense of satisfaction in doing so.

And I can't accept that it doesn't help him to talk. My whole philosophy of life is about emotional authenticity, about processing whatever happens, about looking everything in the face, and knowing it for what it is. He can't understand why anyone would want to talk about something that is so upsetting. For him, a problem shared is a problem doubled. The truth is that, trapped in this tunnel of pain, his needs and mine are diametrically opposed.

We feel like lepers. People see death in our eyes, feel it in the touch of our hands and hurry away. Occasionally people do make oblique suggestions that are intended to be helpful. Camomile tea, acupuncture, a witch who will contact Laura in the afterlife and reassure us that she is happy.

I nod and smile, say little, rage silently. I don't want any of that. I just want a little space for Laura. I just want her to be seen for a moment. I won't allow her to become the kind of problem which can be solved by an alternative therapist, a chat, a coffee, a hasty rummaging through a handbag for a packet of tissues. I do not want to feel better. If I can feel better then she can't have been worth so very much.

I have a coffee with a woman we know who has a badly disabled daughter, expecting her to offer some insight but all she says is – waterproof mascara. I think that's what I've found most helpful. An old school friend who has suffered a stillbirth is more helpful. The verb to cope should never be followed by an adverb, she tells me. You don't cope well or badly. If you're all still alive at the end of the day then that's the most you can expect.

Then I meet up with a Norwegian woman who has suffered not one stillbirth, but two. As she enters the Avenue Louise coffee shop I am fascinated by the fact that she is alive, walking, smiling even. How can she still be doing these things? We talk about men. Her experience is the same as mine. Her husband works harder and harder, goes out, refuses to talk. This, she tells me, is just the way men are.

I reached a stage, she says, when I wondered if I should leave him. Because what's the point of being married to someone if you can't talk about such an important thing? But I still love him. And so now I go and see a shrink every week and that's where I talk about my lost babies. That's the choice I've had to make.

It's a big compromise, I say.

Yes, she says. A very big compromise. But then if you want to keep your marriage together you do have to make some big compromises, I suppose.

We're both silent. And I know we're thinking of all those other women who are also making big compromises. The women married to men who drink, who are unfaithful, never help with the children. And the men who put up with wives who are bitchy, critical, resentful. For this is the landscape of marriage now that we're no longer young. The honeymoons are long gone. Her position and mine may be more extreme than the situation of others but we're far from the only ones making unacceptable compromises.

For a while there's silence and then she says – The main thing that I understand is that this happened to me. It didn't happen to someone else.

I'm mystified by this statement, wonder if she's failing to express herself clearly even though she speaks English as though it's her mother tongue. We move on and finally admit to the worst of all this.

Why doesn't anybody say anything? I ask her, suddenly engulfed in tears.

They won't, she says. They just won't.

I can survive her death, I say. But not the silence.

I know, she says. My babies never had their place, they were never noticed and they never will be now.

We stare at each other, both soaked in tears, as the coffee machine rattles and a waiter starts to offer *tarte tatin* or *mille-feuille* and shuffles away. Both of us are desperate for some enlightenment but none emerges.

I'm endlessly waiting for it all to feel a bit better, I say.

She suggests that I stop waiting. I mention waterproof mascara. Chanel is apparently the only one which definitely won't run – and it comes in several different colours. But I decide that there must be an answer beyond cosmetics. And so I make a promise to Laura – *No one else who is grieving or in pain is going to be left to struggle alone if I can do anything to help them.* Perhaps I won't save the world but I can befriend the suffering. This, at least, provides me with some purpose.

Everyone tells me the same Buddhist story. It is that one about the woman whose child dies and she is so wracked by grief that she goes to the Buddha to ask him to bring the child back to life. The Buddha says that he will grant her wish if she can bring him five mustard seeds from a house in which there has been no death.

The grieving mother immediately sets out to find such a house. She goes from one door to the next asking at each house. Her search goes on for years, she knocks at the door of hundreds, thousands of houses but she can find no house untouched by death. Finally she has to accept that death is a part of human life and so her grief is at an end. Doubtless at that point she also becomes a Buddhist as well.

This story really annoys me. Or perhaps it isn't the story that annoys me but the way it is told. In my world, it seems to be a polite way of saying – difficult things happen to everyone so why don't you forget about it and move on?

I myself don't understand the story in that way. I suspect that the grieving woman was not really as stupid as is suggested. She knew from the beginning that she wouldn't find a house where no one had died. But nevertheless, she felt a need to go to all those houses, to share all those stories. I imagine her sitting at one hundred kitchen tables, listening, talking, crying. To me the story is about the fact that grief is a process and – regrettably, significantly – there are no short cuts.

Every weekend I go to the Quaker Meeting House. I don't know what I'm doing there. I am too selfish, too materialistic, too impatient to be a proper Quaker. In the silence of the Meeting, when I should be waiting for the presence of God, I'm worrying about where I've put that Spider-Man costume that Thomas needs for his party at nursery. But at least at the Meeting House no one tells me to look on the bright side, or count my blessings.

Soon I am asked to join a discussion group which takes place in the evening. It is run by an elderly man called Jack who is partly Irish and partly Scandinavian and his French wife Aurélie. The group meets at their flat which is high and looks out over the St Gilles Hôtel de Ville, the night-time city. Perhaps now I will discover what people at the Meeting House actually believe.

Oh you won't find that out, Jack tells me. For the Quakers, God is a verb. No one really cares what anyone believes, only what they do.

If Jack were thirty years younger, I'd be madly in love with him. And you? I ask. Is that how it works for you?

Jack explains that he identifies himself as a practising non-believer.

When I was in my twenties, he says, I read the Gospels and didn't believe a word of them. But I did think that the life of Christ provides an admirable guide to the way a life should be lived and so that has always been my guide. Then eventually I became a Quaker so that I could continue to pursue that idea without having to accept any particular beliefs. I think one has to live as though it is true.

I ask Jack about my strange experiences in isolated places, the west coast of Wales, what it was that I experienced there. He understands immediately.

Oh yes, he says. I think that does happen. One can be over-whelmed by the sheer there-ness of things. Science can explain so much but I don't think it will ever explain that.

At one of Jack's evening meetings I talk about a woman who wrote on the Sands website that she found the death of her baby beautiful. I had found the comment hard to stomach but had also known, at some level, that her reaction was authentic. Jack considers this and comments that, in the West, we're all of us brought up to make judgements about the things that happen. This is a good day, that was a bad day. This is sad, this is beautiful. But the very act of making all these judgements is exhausting and confusing.

And if even the death of a baby can contain moments of beauty then none of these judgements really have meaning.

Every day is just a day, every event is just an event. Good and evil, ugliness and beauty are so inextricably twisted together that it becomes pointless to try to wrest them apart. No good days, no bad days. Just days. On the rare occasions when I manage to think in this way, I'm much happier. Evil has lost its power – and fear has gone as well.

One November day Thomas and I are heading to Rachel's house after nursery so that Thomas can play with Edie. When we get to the house, Rachel makes me tea and the children disappear into the playroom. Rachel is now heavily pregnant, her baby due within a couple of weeks. They know that the baby will be a boy and they've decided to call him Ethan. After a few moments, Edie appears back in the kitchen, crestfallen.

Mummy, I want to get married to Thomas but he doesn't want to get married to me because he wants to get married to his mummy.

Ah well, Rachel says. I'm sorry, love, but there's a lot of them like that.

When Rachel and I laugh, Edie looks even more distressed and so we take our tea and go through to the playroom, promising to find a game which will cheer her up. Rachel goes to a cupboard to lift a jigsaw down from a high shelf. I see Thomas watching her, his eyes fixed on the tight fabric stretched over her bump. As she moves, we see the baby move inside her.

Rachel, Thomas says. Will your baby die as well?

Rachel doesn't miss a beat, looks him straight in the eyes.

No, love. I don't think so. What happened to your sister was rare and I'm very, very sorry. I don't think the same will happen to our baby.

Thomas seems happy enough with this but he's subdued and his eyes move back to Rachel's belly again and again. I realise that, in this moment, he's come to a new understanding of what happened to his sister. I wish he didn't have to know. A toy drum swings aimlessly from his hand, he doesn't want to do a jigsaw or play at garages. This is how it's going to be – understanding and grieving for him will be long and slow. A process which will last many years, perhaps a lifetime.

The next day Thomas asks me if we have photographs of Laura. I hesitate but decide that it's best to show him the photographs. Get it over with while he's still too young to really know what they mean. So we sit down together and look at the photographs. He's serious, impressed, puzzled rather than upset.

I don't like the ones with no clothes on, he says.

No. I don't either. I want to be able to wrap her up.

Thomas looks through the photographs again and the usual round of questions starts about where she is, why people die. But soon he's forgotten and is busy building an elaborate pulley system to lift his toys, in buckets, up and down the stairwell.

The next day he comes home from nursery and says that he'd like to take the photographs of his sister into nursery for Show And Tell. I don't want to say no but I'm not sure this is appropriate.

I asked my teacher, he says. And she says I can take them in any time.

The next day, when I'm picking him up from nursery, I speak to his teacher. She's a young woman – so young that she looks as though she should still be at school herself. She's Dutch and American, thin, fragile with long red hair and a heart shaped face, bright blue eyes. She wears her hair tied back and dresses in flared jeans, sandals, a shapely T-shirt.

It's fine, she says. Thomas and I have talked and his sister is very important to him so he should bring the photographs in. We can all look at them together.

I'm surprised but put the album of photographs into Thomas's bag. When he comes home, I don't ask what happened because I don't want to make this look like a big issue but later Thomas tells me.

It was good, he says. Everyone sat around and we looked at the photographs. And it was all right most of the time. But then you know those photographs where she hasn't got any clothes on. Well, some of the stupid boys started giggling then.

For a moment, I'm fired with rage. How dare anybody laugh at those photographs? Then I remember that these children are three years old. And what's important about this situation is not the giggles of those bored, small boys but the fact that a young Dutch-American teacher was brave enough to allow the photographs to be shown. Did she not worry that other parents might complain? I'm amazed by her courage. And even the giggles have their purpose. They remind me that not even death can be appalling and magnificent all the time. Sometimes it can be trivial, comic, irrelevant.

At the time of Laura's death we were informed that Stephen's medical insurance covers us for counselling and so I suggest that we book to see a therapist. I've been to see plenty of shrinks before and their waiting rooms always contain the same objects – dusty spider plants and palms, a box of tissues, dated posters of European holiday destinations. I know Stephen considers the counselling a waste of time.

So you had a miscarriage? the counsellor says.

No, Stephen says. No. A stillbirth. It's important to get the words right.

The therapist nods in fake sympathy but thinks we're splitting hairs.

We tell our story and she nods and sighs. And then we leave and go back the next week, and the week after, and talk about it all again and again. Soon long silences develop. The counsellor is becoming frustrated by us.

But your baby is dead, she says to me. She is dead. Then she repeats this statement several times more, as though I am having difficulty understanding.

And if you continue to focus on someone who is dead, she says, then, in some ways, you become dead as well. You can't have a proper relationship with her because she doesn't change or grow. In order to live fully you need to move on.

Beside me I feel Stephen as a silent knot of rage.

You're wrong, I say. Totally wrong. Of course you can have a relationship with someone who is dead. In fact, you have one whether you want it or not. Even after someone has been dead thirty years they still have an influence on your life.

The counsellor smiles and raises her hands as if to fend me off. That may be possible, she says, if you have known someone well over a period of years.

You think we don't know anything about Laura?

Stephen and I have turned into small, crouching people, with bones made of steel. You could run us over in a ten-ton truck and we wouldn't bruise.

No, let me tell you, I say. We do know about Laura. Laura was very strong. She kicked far earlier than other babies and, even after I'd lost pints of blood, her feet were still beating away inside me. And even after my waters had broken, and there was no hope for her, she was still kicking. And the doctors told me that she would be damaged by the infection but the autopsy revealed that she was a perfectly healthy baby.

Yes, I'm sure she was strong. The counsellor's voice has become squeaky.

And that affects my life, I say. In bad moments I can borrow her courage. And I know you think we should draw a line under what has happened. Well, that may work in a psycho-therapy textbook but it doesn't accord with our real under-standing of what death is and how it works.

I didn't say you can't remember the dead, the counsellor says.

It isn't about memory, Stephen says. Memory implies some-thing static.

My idea of her changes and so our relationship is changed, I say. She can be different things to us at different times.

The counsellor is giving me a look that I can't read. Does she think that I'm a grief-crazed lunatic? Or is that a shadow of humility appearing in her eyes? For myself, I know that I'm painfully sane and simply fighting for the right to grieve. It shocks me that I should have to fight – but so it appears to be. The session is finished and Stephen and I gather up our coats.

Now, another appointment? the counsellor says.

No thank you, Stephen says.

In the car home, Stephen and I dismantle the small, crouched people with the steel bones. At the traffic lights, Stephen reaches over and takes my hand.

Working wonders, this counselling, he says. You and I haven't agreed about much recently but just look at all the things we agreed about today.

A few days later, I go out to our local organic grocery store. It smells of herb tea and cedar wood. I bump into a woman whom I vaguely know. She's a large woman with clear skin and very deep brown eyes. She asks how I am. Usually when people ask that question I just say – I'm fine – and then sidle away. But something tells me it's safe to speak.

Yes, she says. Yes. I had been told.

A silence falls between us. Then she looks me directly in the eyes.

Was she beautiful? she says. Was she really beautiful?

Yes, I say. She was very beautiful.

Oh how I wish I'd seen her. I would so much love to have seen her.

The woman produces a tissue from a large bag that swings on her pushchair handle. She probably says other things but I'm too overwhelmed to hear. She lays a hand briefly on my arm before maneuvering her pushchair on down the aisle.

That woman. She understood, she knew. So many months have passed since Laura's death and nobody has ever asked me what she looked like. No one has ever realised that a person died. But the woman in the grocery store knew. This isn't the first time that a virtual stranger has been of far more use than friends. But why? Perhaps it has to do with the fact that we all find expectation difficult. When a disaster happens, people who are close to the afflicted panic because they know that they must rise to the occasion. Many of them crumble under the pressure, or rebel against the weight of expectation. But nothing is expected of a stranger and so they offer whatever they can freely and move on. I never become friends with the grocery-store-woman, we barely see each other again. The fact that she saw Laura – really saw her – does help. But Laura remains as dead as she has always been.

VII

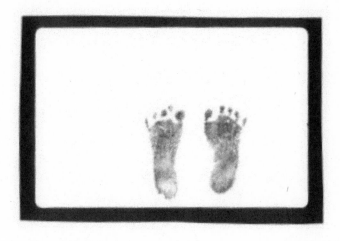

There is no foot too small that it cannot
leave an imprint on the world.

Anonymous

Me-me-me. Moi-moi-moi. Even before Laura died, I didn't have a normal life. My family is truncated, branches are missing. A bolt of lightning struck, a revelation, and now we live blackened and singed. Only the women remain – my mother, my sister and me. My father and my brother have been gone for ten years now and nothing suggests that they will return. My father is on the south coast, in a bungalow overlooking the sea. My brother has gone to Argentina to play polo and I don't even have his address.

I miss them – all the time. A jagged-edged hole gapes where they should be. I think of them more now than I did before. One pain opens up others. But you patch up the gaps, carry on. At least when Laura died there was a funeral and a grave. Losses without graves are more difficult. I have no desire to be a victim. I don't think that my luck is worse than many others. I come from an affluent world and pain does look better when played out against an elegant backdrop.

But still I find myself wanting to know what problems were caused by the Dead Babies and what might have been there anyway. That question can never be answered. In the laboratory of life there is no control sample.

The chronology is breaking down. The screen is beginning to scramble. Periods of time go missing. In fiction, the non-linear narrative is all the fashion but the non-linear life signals only mental disintegration. I open that cardboard box, check my diaries and notebooks. What shocks me is how little I wrote. Those miscarried babies – the later ones don't even have dates. But the first two are there in a few scrawled lines.

Usually I take care never to allow even those first two any

identity. If I think of them at all, I label them only using the short periods of their lives. The first miscarriage is the Easter Baby. The next one, which we lost in the same year, died somewhere in that featureless time around October or November – too late for autumn and too early for Christmas. But still it is the Autumn Baby.

Easter Baby. Autumn Baby. I am entering dangerous territory. Do not allow them any existence. There were too many of them and they came too quickly. It shouldn't be like this, of course. Often when a woman has a miscarriage she gives the baby a name and she marks out the year ahead in terms of should-have-beens. My baby should-have-been in the womb five months by now. Six months, seven, eight.

And the next year it's the same. On this date one year ago we should-have-been. And so on and so on. That is the right and proper process. Grief may lack a landscape, mile markers, distances, but the human mind supplies them. Except that for Stephen and me there are so many dates that I can't afford to remember them all.

Already the year is garlanded by Laura's various anniversaries – the date when we first realised she was in trouble, the date of her death, her due date. And then if one lays on top the dates of the Easter Baby, and allows for an Autumn Baby as well. Life is too short for all that one needs to forget. Did I really lose that year of my life – or did I wilfully mislay it?

In films a miscarriage is dramatic. It involves an elegant woman at a social event in a white dress, suddenly stumbling, a champagne glass dropping from her hand, as a dribble of blood drips down her leg over the strap of her jewelled sandal. And then she faints and the whole of the white dress is soaked in blood. An ambulance is called, panic and distress, a beautiful white face against even whiter hospital sheets, concerned relatives standing around.

My experience of miscarriage is nothing like that. For me, it takes place in slow motion, is dreary rather than dramatic. It involves endless visits to the hospital, bleeding, measuring of the baby. Nothing we can do. Come back in two weeks. Another two weeks. We're not quite sure. Let's wait and see. No heartbeat. No, I'm sorry. Nothing we can do. We're not quite sure. Nothing we can do. Like an old-fashioned record player, the needle stuck in a groove. The same thread of melody playing again and again.

In a notebook I find a date. The 13th of March, 2006. Ten months since Laura's death and the day when the Serb tyrant President Milosevic died. Our friend, Mark James, the BBC Brussels correspondent, is having lunch with us and tells us the news. And in that same instant I know that I am pregnant. Not just another late period. Definitely pregnant because although I feel sick, I'm starting on my third helping of lasagne and my hands are shaking so badly that I have to concentrate to get my fork to my mouth. The beginning of the Easter Baby.

Mark has to leave for The Hague immediately. Stephen is also rushing Thomas and me because in half an hour we're leaving to go to a party at the house of one of his American colleagues. But still I dash out to the Rue du Bailli and buy a pregnancy test kit. Although spring should be starting the air is white with frozen mist. When I arrive back Thomas greets me at the door. Mummy, you know astronauts, they have those special helmets and that's because the air is different on the moon. Why is it different?

Just give me a minute, Thomas, and I'll explain.

I hurry up the stairs and into the loo. My fingers fumble to open the plastic, the stick drops from the package, I catch it, then drop it again and it slides down the loo. Twenty euros down the drain – literally. I consider going out to get another but what's the point? Because I know. I decide not to tell Stephen because I don't want to upset him. I'll wait until the evening when Thomas has gone to bed. I go downstairs and find Stephen with a children's science encyclopedia open on the table, answering questions about the air on the moon.

What else do I remember about the Easter Baby? The Prince of Wales Hotel in Southport: red-brick and Victorian with turrets, gables, an ornate iron portico and a revolving door. We go there for the wedding of one of Stephen's cousins. A proper seaside hotel. I am in heaven. Upstairs is a world of creaky floorboards, frosted glass, patterned carpets and porters in maroon nylon jackets with gold buttons. The smell of gravy rises up through rubbish shafts.

Stephen's family arrive and his father kisses me because he's heard that I'm pregnant again. I wish that no one had been told. Then an aunt I don't know congratulates me as well.

I don't know, I say. I'm not sure.

Oh no, she says. No. It couldn't happen again. It couldn't.

But she may be wrong because this pregnancy increasingly feels similar to the Laura pregnancy. I'm not comfortable. A weight presses on my lower back and my hips. When I sneeze, everything pulls. I have to roll over onto my side before getting out of bed.

The next morning Thomas wakes at six, and Stephen wants to sleep, so I have no choice but to walk. As I manoeuvre the pushchair out through the revolving door, low clouds scurry through glowering skies. Southport is a place of crazy golf and amusement arcades still shut down for the winter. The skeleton outline of a funfair gives the seafront the melancholy look of an industrial wasteland.

The morning is brisk and jewel-bright. Thomas and I can't find the sea – how strange to mislay the sea – but we wander around an inland boating lake where geese paddle amidst stray plastic bags. An elegant little Victorian pavilion with dusty glass has been roughly covered in bright green paint. Despite the fact that I feel headachy, nauseous and hungry, I'm ridiculously happy. Sea salt air and morning sickness mix surprisingly well.

I watch Thomas as he runs away from me around the ornamental boating lake. He is tiny in his navy duffle coat, Thomas the Tank Engine blue woolly hat, corduroy trousers falling down. When he returns to me his eyes are such a striking blue and so very clear. I have always known that without a doubt it was a crime to bring him into the world. I can hardly bear to look at the whiteness of his skin that will bruise so easily.

Now he drags me towards the green-painted pavilion. I sit down on a bench inside, staring out through the dusty windows. He starts to play at shops, selling me the contents of the basket at the bottom of the pushchair: a bottle of water, a packet of wipes, a broken plastic car. As he bends to gather his wares, his Thomas the Tank Engine hat falls off and I reach to pick it up. And feel a spasm inside me, a brief moment of shock, a tightening of muscles. For a moment I think – *that's it, the baby is dead* – then I tell myself to stop being stupid and pull Thomas's hat back onto his head.

Back in Brussels, we go to see Dr Vermeulen at the Hospital of St Clare. Initially she does a scan in her office but then says she needs better equipment and I'm asked to move to another room across the corridor. I should see trouble coming but don't. We're now in the room where they told me that Laura would die.

I don't look at the images on the screen. The news doesn't come as a surprise. I'd expected bad news, but not such bad news. Dr Vermeulen is brisk. I'm beginning to understand the medical profession. They hate what they can't understand. Dr Vermeulen tells me that the baby has been dead for four or five days. I think back – that early morning walk in Southport. So, in the midst of that morning of happiness, a life had ended.

The following day I'm booked in for a D and C, a 'Dilation and Curettage', a procedure for cleaning out the uterus after a miscarriage. Strangely I'm still feeling sick, the body continues its processes even though the purpose of the process has ceased. Inside I feel relatively calm. The publishers are sending the proofs of my book back to me so I need to get home and work on them. I feel guilty that I can't feel more. A human life has been lost, after all. But I'm already worn out by grief. You can't care so much about everything.

A nurse talks about The Intervention and Removing the Post Pregnancy Material. Doubtless they think that euphemisms of this kind are helpful. I wait in a hospital room for hours without food or water. How can I still be ravenously hungry when the baby is dead? As they take me down to the operating theatre, I'm crying because I don't want them to take my baby from me. The people in operating theatres are car mechanics. A few lengths of tubing, nuts and bolts, a metal implement to dig and twist, a bit of mess to clear up. What would a kind word cost them?

The anaesthetist says – Enjoy.

Clamp the mask on, spread my legs, stick some metal implement up inside me, hook the baby out, cut it up to do some tests and then put it in the hospital rubbish. And then I'm back on the road again. And they take me upstairs. My head is fuzzy from the anaesthetic. A nurse arrives and sees my tears.

You've got one child who is alive, she says. That makes you very lucky. Some women aren't able to have any children at all. You need to think positive.

My continuing tears seem to send her into a panic. She suggests to another nurse that the hospital psychologist should be called. I have entered an Alice in Wonderland world. Dr Vermeulen arrives. The intervention was a success, she says. I got it out whole – and not too much bleeding.

I wonder if I'm expected to offer my congratulations.

Of course, you'll have to leave it three months, she says. Before trying to have another. But no longer than that. Time isn't on your side.

Just like a box of chocolates. If you can't have the orange cream you can always have the chocolate truffle instead. I pull my clothes on and leave the hospital. At least I have three months ahead when I don't have to think about pregnancy. I can't go home because Thomas is there and I don't want him to see me crying. Rachel will be looking after baby Ethan. I don't know who to call. I just want to find some place where I can sit quietly and cry but there isn't anywhere. So instead I walk through the city, for miles and miles. I know that I shouldn't be doing this but I can't stop myself. If I keep on the move then I might eventually arrive at a place where this isn't happening.

Inside my head I play a game that I call The Leagues of Grief. It's about trying to work out just how bad what has happened is. How does it compare to the suffering of other people that

I know? The Norwegian mother of those two stillborn babies is definitely in a worse situation than me. I also know of a family who only have one little boy and he's badly disabled. So again that's worse than me.

But most other people I know seem somehow to be better off. They may have had a stillborn baby but they've gone on to have other living children. Maybe I never will. But what's the point of this? Why do I go through all this in my head again and again? Of course, it has to do with the question of entitlement. How much grief am I really entitled to? Of course, I know quite well that the words Grief and Entitlement should never appear in the same sentence. Some people lose a brother and don't really care. Others mourn a cat for twenty years. You just feel what you feel. But still the game goes on.

At the beginning, we should be given a catalogue of all the pain and grief we will have to bear. The catalogue should set it all out in detail: the bereavements and illnesses, the failures and losses. If we had such a schedule then we would be able to apportion grief in proper amounts at proper times.

Now I look back on events in my past, such as splitting up with my first boyfriend, and regret that I allowed it to upset me as it did. I seem to remember spending night after night crying through the small hours. Now it seems to me scandalous that I wasted so much time. Had I known then what greater pains I would have to bear, I would have saved my tears for a real disaster.

And, of course, the worst is definitely yet to come. For me, now that I am approaching forty, the main change I notice is that bad things have started to happen to friends. Evil illnesses, the death of a parent, financial disaster, cancer.

Perhaps I should lay aside some of my grief about Laura, keep it in reserve for whatever else may be coming my way.

At the Quaker discussion group I am told that the Bible contains an important mistranslation. Apparently Christ on the cross did not say – *My God, my God, why hast thou forsaken me?* Instead he said – *My God, my God, for what hast thou forsaken me?* This, I am told, means that we shouldn't bother to ask why people suffer, only what purpose can be found in their suffering.

Later Jack also says – Isn't it strange that the words God and good are so very similar? Only one letter difference. My idea is that maybe two thousand years of European history have been based on a typographical error. There never was any God, only good. Wouldn't it be so much better if that were true? Because no one can work out what God is but everyone knows goodness when they see it.

In two weeks' time it will be the anniversary of Laura's death. I prepare for the date fast and furiously. It's as though Laura is alive and I'm wrapping the presents, making the cake, sending out the invitations for the party. But instead Thomas and I are making a box so I can put all of her things in it. Of course, she doesn't actually have any things but there are a few letters and cards I should keep.

The day before the anniversary I go down into the centre of town and have Laura's name and her one date tattooed onto my foot. Although I am not a tattoo kind of person, I've always liked the idea of something that is permanently part of the human body. Now she'll be with me every time I put my foot to the ground.

That evening I go to the Quaker discussion group and take my photographs of Laura. People pass the photographs around and Jack lights a candle. As so often before, we get into a conversation about the human need to ascribe meaning to events which are, in reality, entirely random. Samuel Hayden says – Of course Nietzsche was right when he said that God is dead. He is dead. Because nowadays we don't want someone to tell us the meaning of a certain thing, we want to find that meaning out for ourselves. We have taken over the role of creation and we are all Gods now.

I think about the box and the tattoo. Perhaps they're my attempt at meaning.

Late that night I wake and can't get back to sleep. I creep down through the dark house, put the light on in Stephen's study, switch on the computer. I read some messages on the forum and then click on the chat room button. I've never used a computer chat room before but it's easy to see how it works.

Only one other person is online. A twenty-two-year-old from Matlock called Dave. He's typing from the computer in his dad's garage. His son Johnny was stillborn three months ago, he writes. So perfect but he never breathed and no one can explain why. Dave works in the catering industry but he has to keep going out into the back yard, and hiding behind the bins, because he can't stop crying. At the weekend he likes to visit Johnny's grave but his mother-in-law has told him that he shouldn't waste his time. He's barely on speaking terms with his wife because she wants to try for a new baby straightaway but Dave doesn't want another baby ever. He is Johnny's dad and that's enough for him.

I type – I am so very, very sorry. Then I type it again and again and again. After that I hold my finger down on the open brackets button and then on the closed brackets button. I know from reading the forum that brackets are the online symbol for a hug. As I do so, I ask myself what value a few symbols appearing on a computer screen can possibly have. But Dave thanks me very much and we 'talk' for a while longer. Dave promises to light a candle for Laura in the church near where he works. Somehow the idea of that candle burning far away in Matlock, and the thought of Dave's courage – as he cries behind the bins – makes the thought of her anniversary possible.

The day dawns and it doesn't look so bad. It turns out that the idea of the anniversary was the problem, not the anniversary itself. Stephen and I have made an agreement that we'll always take a day off on Laura's birthday. This year I wanted to go to the coast but Stephen feels he's done too many wind-swept seafronts recently and so we've booked to go to Paris for the day by train. Big Alice has kindly agreed to pick Thomas up from nursery for us.

In Paris it's raining – that particular kind of Parisian rain which is wetter than other rains – but we head to Le Marais and find a place to have lunch: a café with red-and-white-checked tablecloths. We're both of us conscious of the time. We'll know when it reaches the exact moment at which she was born. We sit in silence for a while, with the rain beating down, and people skittering past with umbrellas. One man is holding a newspaper over his head. Somewhere a siren blares. The waiter is rude, the food divine.

Well, at least what's happening this year isn't as bad as what happened this time last year, I say, and Stephen agrees.

Afterwards we walk back to the Gare du Nord under an umbrella. On the way we pass a kitchen shop and I buy a spatula, the kind one uses to get a fried egg out of a pan. The plastic part of it is turquoise and I have it still, although the edge of it is brown now and cracked. I realise that we've been waiting and waiting. And now that this deadline has passed we'll be waiting again – but for what?

I'm getting better now, I know I am. The main characteristic of fresh grief is that it is entirely selfish. You don't want to hear about anyone else's problems, you don't want to listen to other people's stories. You are the only person who has ever lost anyone and your loss is bigger and more terrible than anyone else's. This mode of thinking persists for some time. It is a highly unattractive state in which to live.

Then one day you realise that something has shifted. You look up at the sky and you see all the stars and it seems that each star represents an individual loss. And the more you look, the more there are. They stretch away endlessly into the blackness, hundreds and thousands, far beyond number. And your own particular pain becomes just one tiny prick of light in that vast and intricate tapestry of human loss. You know then that you're on your way back to the world.

It's Stephen and my fifth wedding anniversary. Mum and my West London aunt have offered to look after Thomas so we can have a night away together. A for Anderlecht, B for Boitsfort, C for Châtelain, D for Death, E for Eastbourne – a place we have not visited before. The coastline here is more interesting than Brighton, more shapely and undulating, with a steeper drop to the sea. And there is none of the razzamatazz of Brighton, instead just rows of stately white hotels. Everything is slow and sedate and the few entertainment arcades and seaside sweet shops have already shut up at six o'clock as we walk on the pier.

We stay in the Grand Hotel, a place of towering white pillars and equally vast potted palms. In the morning we wake to a sea which is grey-brown and a tide so high that its restless mass of water seems perilously close to the sedate seafront. The water is choppy rather than rough, heaving and swelling, as though some vast animal of the deep is suffering from stomach ache. Nothing as grand as a white horse, more the occasional flicker of dirty lace. And above, the sky is the same colour as the sea, and the rain is coming down with a steady purpose, sideways, across that grey and white scene.

We walk along the seafront towards Beachy Head – a promontory whose drama seems much increased by the fact that it's constantly shrouded in mist. The seafront is edged by chalets, charming little Victorian huts that are more substantial and elegant than the classic beach hut. Then we turn back, and come to the Wish Tower Café, a 1970s tearoom, high up and jutting out over the sea. Huge windows are filled by mist and spray from the sea. Around us are walking sticks, peaked tweed caps and iced buns.

Stephen and I talk about our plans. The first conversation is easy enough. We know that we are going to move back to England at some point. Two years ago, worried by escalating property prices in England, we bought a house in Gloucestershire in preparation for our return. A strange house with a mini tower on it which is now rented out and fast falling into further disrepair. I used to dream of that house often, of the life we would have there. I don't any more. But still we need to decide when exactly we will move there. Brussels has been our home for so long that it is hard to imagine leaving, but finally we decide that Thomas should start school in England by the time he is six – so that leaves us two more years in Brussels.

The next conversation is more difficult. I don't want to try and get pregnant again but I can't tell Stephen that. It seems to me that we have one child and that's enough. Someone is trying to tell us that we are not destined to have a second child and we should listen to them. It's never a good idea to do battle with the inevitable. I want whatever happens.

But I know that Stephen isn't interested in any vague talk of destiny.

We also talk about our isolation, about the people who haven't been in touch with us and whom we have not contacted. I promise to try harder – but I know that I won't. I don't understand the point of human relationships any more. In some stubborn, self-pitying corner of my mind, I feel that since people don't understand about Laura then they don't understand anything, and so there's no point in talking to them at all. For Stephen, it's different. He feels Laura's death as deeply as I do – probably more so – but he can put it in a box and carry on with other things in his life. He still wants a social life, friends.

I do see some people, I say.

Yes, he agrees. But only people who are also in some sort of trouble. Of course, it's a good thing for you to help other people. Of course. But you do rather pick them. Couldn't we have some normal friends as well?

Fifty per cent of marriages don't survive the death of a baby. I can see now how easily you can slip to the wrong side of that line. Both he and I want to begin again, but the only way we can really do that is by getting away from the memories, and that means getting away from the only other person who was there. Grief is all that's holding our marriage together.

VIII

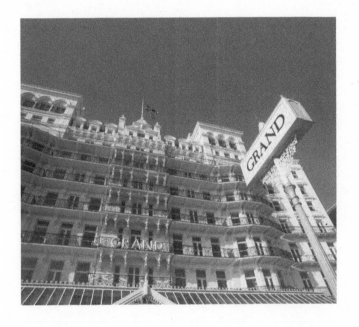

Anger is a bridge across the abyss of loss.

Christine Jette

Another thing I don't like about memoirs: they aren't accounts of a whole life, they can't be. As with a novel, the process of writing a memoir turns out to be largely about identifying the stories you are not going to tell, closing doors, limiting the field of vision rather than expanding it. We all have a number of different lives that run concurrently. We are colleagues, employers, wives, mothers, customers. Anyone who attempts to record all this finishes up with the muddle that is the present moment. Events need to be selected and shaped, themes must run through the narrative. A book is an echo chamber – it depends on repetition, resonance.

I could have written about how I lost my father and brother. Or recorded the experience of being an expat for sixteen years. But instead I've chosen to write about our daughter's death and the events that followed. That makes it seem as though everything during that time was about Dead Babies. I could, however, write a very different account of that time and it wouldn't be a lie. But the choice I have made is Dead Babies and so I need to stick to that.

And, in truth, death was the distinguishing feature of that time. Tragedy attracts tragedy. You enter a cramped and grey town called Tragedy-ville, with endless boarded-up shops, ring roads and dead ends, and you can't find the way out. The only people you meet in that town are other members of the Bereavement Club. You see only difficulty and pain. People dump their bad news on you because they feel that you will understand. That's how it works. But remember, as the Russians say, no one lies like an eyewitness.

I knew from the beginning that the Autumn Baby wouldn't last. Paradoxically this was because I didn't feel nearly as ill as I would usually have done. I lost a few drops of blood and I felt strange pains, but I couldn't trust myself any longer. Maybe the pains were in my imagination? I didn't go to the hospital – although the few people I told urged me to – because I knew they could do nothing. And I felt that, if I kept away from the hospital, then I couldn't be told any bad news. Instead I made myself busy writing my new book. Put the washing machine on, hang clothes on the line, load the dishwasher, rewrite that rambling second chapter, help Thomas to make a crocodile out of egg boxes painted green.

The rest I can't remember – except the hospital. Scans, measuring, bleeding. I'm not sure. No, I'm sorry. Nothing we can do. Then the operating theatre again. Everything is machines, tubes, monitors, flashing lights, concrete floors, no windows. Everyone wears a mask. It's cold as a fridge. I cease to be a human being – and the staff ceased to be human beings a long time ago. After I come around from the anaesthetic, I find myself in a large underground room, with people in other beds ranged around the walls. Some distance away green-clad nurses gather around a central desk.

I start to shake and soon I'm leaping up and down on the bed. I try to call out but my mouth doesn't work. In the distance two nurses are looking at a packet of photographs, giggling. My mouth is opening and shutting and inside I'm screaming, but no noise is coming out. I assume that this is just a bad reaction to the anaesthetic but I don't know. Please, please will someone come? I'm falling off the bed now and my convulsing limbs refuse to move me back to safety.

Eventually the nurses look up and slowly put the photographs away. They treat me as though I'm being tiresome. Special blankets are brought. They don't seem to understand that I can't speak. And locked up in my silence, I am more angry than I have ever been before. A needle is stuck in my arm and gradually the shaking stops and my powers of speech return. A nurse adjusts the drip in my arm.

I say – So what do you do with the Dead Babies? Put them in the hospital rubbish?

Yes, she says. We put them in the rubbish.

Then she looks at me and, for the briefest moment, realises that I am human.

We put them in a special rubbish bin, she tells me.

When I wake again I'm back in the hospital room. The grey and pink walls swirl, the lights dazzle. But I am not in as much pain as I was last time. The baby must have been coming away inside me because they haven't cut me as much. Dr Vermeulen appears with a nurse beside her. Safety in numbers. They stand far away, their backs pressed against a section of the wall next to the door. Dr Vermeulen says various things about The Intervention. Both she and the nurse nod their heads like puppets, look grave. I long for them to leave. But then I remember that there is a question that I must ask.

I have a problem, don't I?

Yes, Dr Vermeulen says. Yes, you definitely have a problem. But it isn't something that I can diagnose or treat. Of course, we'll do all the tests in case we can find out anything – but I wouldn't hold out too much hope of an answer. You know, every year the researchers hold a conference where they update people like me on the latest information about recurrent miscarriages. I usually go to the conference but it's a complete waste of time. They understand nothing.

She moves forward from the wall, just a step.

You need to focus on the child you have, she says. Of course, to have another child would make a – how can I say? A fuller family.

I try to focus my gaze on her but she mixes with the pink and grey of the wall.

She takes another step forward.

I do understand, she says. I lost a baby at twenty-eight weeks myself. Others as well.

I look at her in disbelief. Why has it taken her this long to tell me this information? She understands what is happening to me and yet she has chosen not to speak? And now she looks as though she regrets speaking, backs out of the door, mumbling something about how one child is already enough. The nurse stays, goes in on the attack. *Think positive. Be grateful for what you have.* I shut my eyes and ears. *We put your baby in the hospital rubbish. No need to make a fuss. A special rubbish bin.*

When I open my eyes, the nurse has gone. I need to leave the hospital immediately. It isn't possible for me to stay a moment longer. The hospital is dangerous, my life is at risk. I start trying to put my clothes on but there is a plastic tube in my arm. I rip off translucent tape, pull at the tube, watch the blood-covered thread come sliding out of the cut in my arm.

I know that I am behaving unreasonably. But I am in the land of unreason and feel gloriously liberated. I can do whatever I want now. I pull my clothes on and set off down the corridor, trying to ignore the blood that is spilling everywhere. Does a human arm really contain this much blood? Maybe I should look for a bandage and wrap that round it?

A nurse sees me, gasps, disappears. More nurses appear. They try to catch hold of me but I resist. I'm leaving this hospital now. If I don't, then I'll die. But the nurses take hold of me and suddenly everything is spinning and then I'm back in the hospital room, lying on the bed, and the tube is back in my arm.

A different nurse appears and she is kind. Of Asian origin, she's young and pretty with flawless skin and shiny black hair held back by two silver clips. I don't understand much of what she says, only that she is new to nursing, is in the hospital for a short training period. Oh yes, I think. She hasn't yet learnt to be callous.

I know that this isn't fair because these people don't know my history and they deal with situations far worse than mine every day. They do need to have a level of detachment. But none of that is an adequate excuse. I don't expect them to give long speeches of sympathy or to solve my problem. I only want a few words of human kindness.

Thomas has started refusing to go to nursery. It isn't clear why because he likes nursery. But every morning I have to clean his teeth, put on his clothes, feed him his breakfast. Then sometimes I have to pull him wailing down the street. I don't find that difficult. I'm a tough mum, easily able to discipline a tricky child.

But it's when we get to the nursery that the trouble really starts. There he doesn't scream, or kick, or struggle. Instead he is reasonable and sensible, argues his case clearly. I just don't want you to leave, Mummy. It's not right for you to leave. You need to stay here with me. You will be much better here with me.

His teacher is not concerned. She sees it often. Thomas is just going through a phase of insecurity. But then one morning, as we go through the usual conversation outside the classroom door, I bend down to his level to give him a hug and

I look into his clouded little eyes. And I know the teacher is wrong. Thomas isn't worried for himself, he's worried for me. He doesn't want to leave me because he doesn't trust me to look after myself.

This is all wrong. I am meant to look after Thomas, he isn't meant to look after me. I am losing the battle to keep him separate from what is happening. And I'm breaking the promise that Stephen and I made to ourselves when Laura died. Thomas isn't going to pay for what has happened.

But black and white have merged. I can't make simple judgements any more. Perhaps we all reach a stage in our lives when we suddenly understand the failings of our parents, of parents in general. When we see that, however much you might want to be a good mother, you are sometimes defeated by sheer weight of circumstance. But still I'm going to fight for him to be happy, and that means he needs a happy mum.

I go home and make an appointment to see a shrink – a different one. A woman called Helga who works from her home just across the square and has been recommended by a friend. I don't discuss this with Stephen. He has his own process of grief and it doesn't involve shrinks. He is busy taking Thomas to the park, paying the bills, dealing with tax and car insurance. Keeping the whole show on the road. These things are important, they've got to be done – and they are what he can do.

A few weeks later I turn forty and decide to become a member of the Quaker Meeting House. This is a decision which has few practical implications. Some people are Members of the Meeting, some are Attenders. It makes no difference which you are. After this news is announced, an elderly Quaker congratulates me.

Quakerism is like family, he tells me.

I am surprised by this statement as it contains a note of sentimentality which is generally absent at the Meeting House. Perhaps the elderly man reads the look on my face because he quickly explains himself.

No, no, he says. I don't mean family like that. I mean family in the real sense. You know. People who drive you mad, you can't stand them, you disagree with everything they say and you're endlessly longing to get away from them. That sort of family. But still they are the place to which you come home.

Neither Stephen nor I have the energy or interest necessary to organise a celebration for my birthday but we do go away to Brighton for the weekend, leaving Thomas with my West London aunt. The trains are delayed and we finish up on a Rail Replacement bus winding through one unforgiving, nameless suburb after another, queuing again and again at what appears to be the same toxic junction. England is a country that is now quite foreign to us. What did they do with the England of our childhood? When will they give it back to us?

We stay at the Grand Hotel in a room on the fourth floor overlooking the sea. A vicious storm is stirring. I get up at two o'clock in the morning and stand at the window looking out at the sea as it bubbles and heaves, throws itself up against the sea wall. The hotel is creaking and groaning, the roof tiles cling on perilously. The stars are shaking, their fragile lights flickering. I love the power of it, the risk.

Next morning the town is littered with stray dustbin lids, rubbish and twigs. I wander through the Lanes, idly staring into shop windows. I have always entirely rejected the idea of retail therapy, considering it to be for stupid people. And all around me the new mood is anti-consumerism, friends tell me endlessly that they are cutting down on what they buy. As ever, I am out of step, paddling against the tide. I know perfectly well that the right skirt is not going to fix our problem but if it makes me feel better for a day or two then that is enough.

And so I buy myself too many expensive clothes. I justify this by telling myself that I need to take myself in hand. I can't do anything about the Dead Babies but there is no need for me to be fat and badly dressed as well. In our modern society the opposite of pain is not peace but shopping.

IX

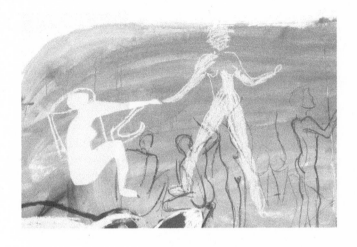

A son is a son until he takes a wife.
A daughter is a daughter for the rest of your life.

Anonymous / Traditional

What exactly is a miscarriage? Perhaps it's just a heavy period, the loss of a few cells. After all, as many as 50 per cent of pregnancies may end in a miscarriage in the early stages. Sometimes a woman doesn't even know that she has miscarried. In the past, before the era of scans, a woman wasn't considered to be pregnant until she had missed three periods. For women in most of the world, that continues to be the case.

So a miscarriage is nothing.

And everything.

Because a life which could be happening isn't happening. A person is absent, missing. And that particular, unique life will not come again. And here in the Western world, where scanning is routine, the mother will have heard a heartbeat, or seen a shape on a screen. She will have begun to hope, dream, plan. She will have been bombarded with marketing literature showing her pictures of the family she will soon have. What she loses is a dream, an idea, a future. And that can be harder to bear than many more concrete losses.

Everything and nothing. Now you see me, now you don't. Just a few cells. An everyday loss but it's the very fact that it's ordinary which makes it devastating. No woman who has a miscarriage will ever forget. Many women live forever with a shadow baby. When their six-year-old and two-year-old walk away down the road, the four-year-old that never was goes with them. A miscarriage isn't Zimbabwe or the Horn of Africa. Nothing like as bad as stillbirth. But there aren't any easy ways to lose a baby.

The summer may have come. I have no memory of it, my notebooks and diaries reveal nothing. I put the washing machine on, hang clothes on the line, load the dishwasher, write a one-act play, tell Thomas – yet again – that spitting in cake mixture is not acceptable. The truth is that anyone can survive a crisis. It's the daily grind that kills. On death certificates it says – cancer, stroke, heart attack. It never says – she just opened the fridge and, when confronted yet again with the task of turning four cold sausages and a lump of cheddar into a tasty family supper, she simply lay down and died. But nevertheless I am sure that tragedy is less likely to kill than domestic boredom.

Then – and this is definitely recorded in my diary – I meet Joslin. I see her first at the Quaker Meeting House – spot her across a crowded room and fall for her. Tall and blonde, she wears a scarf tied in her hair and a long gathered skirt. She has an odd simplicity and gladness to her, like some scrubbed-clean East German peasant in one of those Soviet posters insisting on the wholesome happiness of the communist regime. Her children, Ellie and James, white-blonde and luminous, hold onto her hands.

I've rather forgotten how to do friends, I tell her.

I'm going to make you remember.

Joslin is clever, thoughtful, honest. A person of tireless energy, endless resources. She invites me around to her house and so, after I've picked Thomas up from nursery, we board the tram and travel to St Josse. Joslin lives in a tall Belgian town house, similar to ours, to so many others in this city. The exterior is both forbidding and bland but, inside, the house is light with ten-foot ceilings, marble fireplaces, each room opening into another through heavy double doors. Joslin makes tea and the children get out plasticene and paints.

I'm not going to pretend to you that I can possibly imagine what it must be like to live without Laura, she says. But I'm going to try. I really am. Also I'm just going to say whatever I think about grief and all that. You'll just have to accept that loads of it will be tactless and inappropriate. I reckon that's still better than saying nothing, don't you?

Joslin organises the children with their paints.

If you have to go to the hospital, she says, I'll come with you. You mustn't deal with those people on your own.

The kindness of this offer nearly reduces me to tears.

I talk to her about the experience of taking Clomid and Utrogestan, drugs I've been prescribed which are meant to increase the chances that I'll get pregnant and keep the baby. She already knows about that because she was given Clomid when she couldn't get pregnant.

That drug made me mad, she says. Raving mad.

I know. The other day I finished up kicking the car and screaming.

Exactly, she says. It's dangerous. These doctors have no idea what they're prescribing. But the point is – that's the drug, not you.

I am unconvinced. The drugs may be exacerbating the situation but I know that, even before, I was losing my grip.

The next step is IVF, I tell her.

So, will you do that?

I don't know. Stephen thinks we should, so does my mum.

And you?

IVF is a treatment for people who can't get pregnant. I've been pregnant three times in the last two years so what's it going to do for me?

The children are bored with painting now so Joslin puts on music and dances with them, falls in love with Thomas.

You know he's something special, don't you?

You don't have to tell me that because he's the only one.

I'm not. It's just what I think.

Soon I find myself going to Joslin's house nearly every day. She is an artist and she shows me some of her work. Before she was married, she worked with a group of other women artists and they took off all their clothes, covered themselves in paint, rolled around on giant sheets of paper. She shows me the resulting images. They are both massive and partial, dislocated, elusive. Like Henry Moore sculptures but with a feminine grace and fluidity.

She says little about her husband. I know his reputation and wonder how she came to be married to such a man. She carries on regardless, refuses to allow anything that he does to touch the graceful lives she makes for herself and her children. Only once she says – The strange thing is that I could tell you a story about my marriage and it would all sound so lovely and you'd think – aren't they a beautiful couple? And I could tell you another story and you'd think – I don't give that marriage long. But the strange thing is that neither story would be a lie.

I love Joslin but I'm also nervous of her. She tells me quite openly that she used to suffer from serious depression. Having suffered from that condition myself, I have no sympathy for depressives. I'm frightened of having to deal with that deep gloom which never shifts, which drags everything and everyone into darkness.

I know my history frightens people, she says. But I'm not like that any more. And it turns out to be true. Instead, Joslin has a simple plan for dealing with her own misery and with that of others.

When I arrive at her house she often says – I'm so fed up. Is it OK if I just spend ten minutes telling you how bad I feel?

But only ten minutes and then after that we'll talk about something else. OK?

I agree and it works just as she says. For ten minutes she rants, moans, complains, bitches. Husband, kids, frustration at lack of time to make her work, her awful parents, mess in the house. And then the ten minutes ends.

OK. Enough. Let's talk about something else.

And the afternoon brightens.

Sometimes she says to me – Go on. Take ten minutes. And remember, you can be as self-indulgent and spiteful as you want.

And so for ten minutes it all comes out. The latest round of tactless comments, my hatred of the medical profession, domestic resentment, bitterness about other women and their living babies. But by the time the ten minutes is up, I'm beginning to laugh at the things I'm saying and at myself. So very simple and yet it works.

I also talk to Joslin about Thomas. I worry about him because he's too good to be true. He's charming, funny, everyone loves him, the nursery can't stop telling me how wonderful he is, when we play games together he throws six after six after six. Is this the child he really is? Or is this the child he has had to become because of his sister's death, because he has no living sibling?

It's getting worse all the time, I say to Joslin. Each time we lose another he becomes more of a miracle. In my mind he has become The One That Got Away. It's increasingly clear that I'm a woman who can't really carry a child and yet I did carry him. But I just want him to be a normal little boy. I don't want him to have to be a miracle, a star.

I don't think you can do anything about it, Joslin says. That's the role he was born to whether you like it or not. At least, thank God, he is naturally an All Singing, All Dancing child. Imagine if he was painfully shy and solitary – now that would be hard for him.

As we head home from Joslin's house I ask Thomas what he feels.

I don't know, he says, as we sit side by side in the tram. But Mummy, I don't really think you should have another baby. The thing is you're not really very good at coping with me so I don't think you'd do well with another.

He opens some cake wrapped in tin foil that Joslin gave him to eat on the way home. It's dark outside, the lights of the city fractured by the dusty windows of the tram. Briefly we catch sight of men sitting outside a bar, drinking, huddled beside heaters, their glasses raised in a toast, their faces lit with brief, radiant smiles. People are crammed in all around us – weary end-of-day office faces and elderly ladies clutching small dogs in knitted jackets. The tram turns a corner and Thomas leans into me, munching cake. Then he puts his hand up into my hair, chews and swallows.

But sometimes, he says, I do find it difficult being all of your children.

I love Joslin and I hate her. The hate comes from jealousy because she is the person I would like to be – and am not. She buys all her clothes in second-hand shops but always looks stunning. She never puts her children in front of a DVD with a plate of chocolate biscuits. She knows all her neighbours and looks after their children. She takes trouble with people, she is good, genuinely good, in a way that I am not.

So many late afternoons spent sitting in her house, with the rain coming down. That Belgian rain which falls endlessly, seeps into everything, envelops the whole city in a thick, bone-soaking mist. The trams, the blackened buildings, the Arab corner shops, the park railings. The children play and we drink tea, talk about what it means to be here and now. Past the honeymoon, exhausted by children and their mess, wondering what happened to the girls we were only a few years before.

We also talk about Quakerism. Joslin is an atheist and her family would be furious if they thought she'd become involved in any kind of spiritual movement.

When I first went to the Meeting House I told them I don't believe any of that religious stuff, she says. But no one was really interested. Apparently there's a whole group of Quaker atheists.

But then what do you want out of it?

I suppose a structure, an idea about how to live. And I want the children to think about these things. To have those values. I don't know.

I admit that I also don't know but tell her about the various strange experiences I have, such as that morning in West Wales. The other occasions when I have been overwhelmed and frightened by the certainty of a great presence so that now I've come to avoid lonely and isolated places for fear of what might happen there.

She is – rightly – dismissive.

No. That's not God. It's just you being neurotic.

We both of us laugh while knowing that there is a larger conversation which we are avoiding.

If God is meant to be within us, Joslin says, then which bit of us is He? Maybe the bit that can imagine how things might be better?

I remember this conversation when, a week later, I find Joslin uncharacteristically deflated, morose. I make the tea and she sinks into a chair and says – Oh for Christ's sake. What's the matter with women like you and me? Why are we always trying to improve everything? We can't look at a child without wanting to engage it in a worthwhile craft project. We can't see a garden without wanting to weed it. We worry that the carrots aren't organic, the thank you card isn't written. We can barely approach the fridge because we're so wracked with guilt about the past-their-sell-by-date yoghurts we'll have to throw in the bin. If this is God, then He's very tiring.

I know – and all this improvement just makes us unhappy.

Yeah, that's my point. Wouldn't it be better just to say – this is it? To see God as the bit of us that knows that it's not going to get any better. We're never going to be slimmer, or have tidier houses, or do more yoga. Our children are not going to watch less television.

We both of us agree to try to give up on improvement – and fail.

Now when I think of Joslin I ask – at some level did I know? Did I see the marks on her? I certainly knew that she, like me, is someone to whom things happen. But no, I didn't see it and neither did she. If there were signposts, omens, warnings, we failed to notice them. We were just two people who met on a steep and rocky section of the path, fell into step. Neither of us had any idea of what was waiting, over the hill, round the next bend.

X

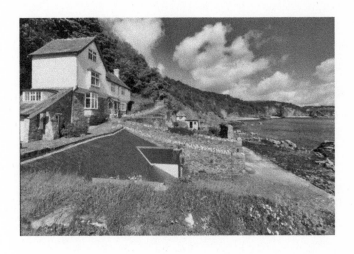

When we arrive at the pearly gates, God will
ask us to account for every hour
not spent by the sea.

Anonymous

When you write a novel it's important to have a strong protagonist with a clear mission or goal. This is advice that agents, publishers, books about creative writing, always give. I may even have said this to my students on occasions. But this advice raises a problem for the writer who aims to record the truth because in real life many women – and men – are neither strong nor purposeful.

But how tempting now to follow that simplistic advice, to present myself as decisive, driven. To make this book into the classic narrative of the quest. *A woman's struggle to have a living second child.* So very simple. But the truth is that I was never sure I wanted another child. I had one lovely son and a daughter – albeit dead – so shouldn't that be enough? It was this that I discussed endlessly with Helga the Shrink, during those many hours in her basement room.

I'm not the motherhood type, I say again and again. Babies bore me. I want to write books, not change nappies. Those maternal types, so brisk and practical, carrying those neat bags with bottles and nappies and wipes and teething gel and pots of mushed up vegetables – I hate them.

Uuum, yes, Helga says, as shrinks do.

And I'm frightened that even if I have a living, second child I'll look at it and think – no, that's not the right baby. And I'm frightened that the child will be a boy. And anyway, I'm forty. One stillbirth, two miscarriages. Isn't it time for me to read the signs?

Uuum. Maybe.

And so I make up my mind again and again that I don't want a second child. But some other part of me won't let go. I've never felt such war within myself. What is this part of me that won't listen to reason? I've always firmly believed that, if we listen carefully enough, then deep down we all know what we need and want. But that's a belief that I'm now being forced to abandon. Later I will realise that often it isn't difficult to know what we want, only difficult to forgive ourselves for what we want.

Dr Vermeulen has suggested that every month we use an ovulation test kit. These kits can be purchased in any chemist and you pee on them first thing in the morning. When they show a red line, that is an indication that you should have sex sometime during the next forty-eight hours. So now that three months have passed since the last miscarriage, I start to use these kits.

We're staying at my aunt's house in West London. I know that the time must be approaching when the stick will show red. I get up in the morning and sure enough, the line is there. But the walls of our bedroom are thin, the bed creaks and Thomas is in the next room. We need to have sex within the next forty-eight hours but Stephen is leaving on a business trip. If we do it quickly now then at least there will be a chance. But it's six o'clock in the morning and both of us are tired and conscious of the creaking bed. I put my arms around Stephen and try to pretend that this is what we want to do. The door slides open.

Daddy, I was wondering if you'd like a game of chess?

Thomas, it's six o'clock in the morning. Go back to bed.

I turn over and then sit up, head in my hands. I'm trying not to cry.

Sorry, Thomas says. Sorry. I'm very sorry.

It's OK, I say through my hands. Darling, it's OK. It's not your fault.

Sorry, Mummy. I'm sorry.

It's OK, Stephen says. It's OK. We can have a game of chess if you fancy that.

Really?

Yes, of course. You go and get the board. Mummy is OK. She just needs a rest.

And so I put my head under the duvet while Stephen plays chess in the half-light of the bedroom with the board balanced on his knees. I don't care so much about the lost opportunity for pregnancy, about the sand running down through the egg timer. But I do care about what's happening to our marriage, about the invasion of those things which are most intimate, the fact that our love now has to run on a timetable. I keep on telling myself that what's happening to us is just bad luck. It doesn't say anything about our worth as people, the quality of our marriage. But it's hard not to conclude that our love has failed.

I listen to the click of the chess pieces on the board, Stephen guiding Thomas through his next possible moves. Around us the streets of West London are slowly waking. Kettles go on, post is picked up from mats, cats are fed. What happens in those other lives? Doubtless there's suffering out there very much worse than ours. This isn't Zimbabwe or the Horn of Africa.

Thomas puts his head against my back. I love you, Mummy.

I love you too, Thomas. How is your life?

It's pretty good, he says. Although I don't much like the lunches.

As the long weeks with Helga pass, I begin to understand, at least to some degree. The story goes like this. Many modern women are in a state of confusion because our society has created opportunities for them beyond reproduction. It's given them education, the possibility of many different kinds of work. But deep down most women still have, in their sub-conscious minds, a primeval instinct which is concerned only with the survival of the species.

And so as a result, the modern woman's attitude to mother-hood is often complicated. But in my case the situation is worse because my body has prepared itself for motherhood several times over but has been disappointed. So now I exist in a state of arrested motherhood and that primeval drive is running out of control.

I remember, years ago, I heard a Radio 4 interview with a woman who had had fourteen miscarriages. At the time I couldn't understand how she could be so stupid. Why didn't she just give up? Now I understand – but the knowledge doesn't change anything. We have become like gamblers who have lost so much that only a win can save them. Good money after bad.

The newspapers are full of the disappearance of Madeleine McCann. Sarkozy takes over from Chirac as President of France. The violence in Iraq continues. The second anniver-sary of Laura's death arrives. It falls on a Saturday so Stephen and I won't be able to have a quiet day together as we did last year. Then I get invited to a book launch in London on that day and decide to go. At the book launch, I'm buzzing with thoughts about writing, plans for the future.

Then a woman says to me – You've got two, haven't you?
No, only the one, sadly.
No. You've got two.
Look. Sorry. I've just said. I've only got——
Books, she says. I'm talking about books.
Oh right. Books.

The hour of three o'clock approaches, but I'm confused. Would it be two or four o'clock in Brussels? And why the hell does it matter anyway? I hurry away from the book launch and try to find a quiet café but everywhere is crowded. Every space full of pushchairs and pregnant women, their vast bellies bouncing up against each other, pressing the air from the room. I squeeze into a corner, thin and trapped.

Later I go out and buy yet more clothes which I don't need. Then I go back to the hotel where I'm staying. I used to have hundreds of friends in London so why am I staying in a hotel? I buy some notepaper and write a letter to Laura. *I miss you and I love you. It's so hard here without you.*

Back in Brussels, Stephen and I go round to the house of friends for supper and meet an Irish couple called Charles and Helen. Stephen knows Charles through work and I have met Helen before but I don't know her. However, I do know her story. In the small world of expatriate Brussels, it is talked of in hushed whispers – as I suppose our own history sometimes is.

Charles and Helen had a little boy and then she got pregnant with a second boy. When she was six months into the pregnancy, it was realised that she is a carrier of a rare genetic disease. That second baby had the disease and was stillborn. They still hoped to have another child but the chances that the disease would recur were high and tests could only be done two months into the pregnancy. Effectively this meant that she had to get pregnant, wait for two months and then have tests. If the disease was present, then she would have an abortion.

Apparently this happened several times over.

In The Leagues of Grief, they score infinitely higher than we do. But then help arrived in the form of a new technology called PGS. This allows an embryo of only two days old to be tested for genetic diseases. As a result, she could do IVF and the doctors would then test the embryos and only implant one that they knew to be in good health. And so Helen finally had a much longed for healthy second child.

I know all this when I meet her at dinner. As the evening wears on we get talking.

I think it's fine to have only one child, she says. It's fine.

I'm surprised but I don't bother to say anything.

Having only one child is fine, she says again.

For me, it's not, I say.

I think it's fine, she says. I don't think you have to worry about it.

I'm beginning to find this conversation both puzzling and offensive.

I'm getting on with my life, I say. But I don't think it's fine.

It is, she says. It is. It's fine to only have one child.

Suddenly she bursts into tears, leaves the table. I wait for a while but then follow her, find her in a distant bedroom. She wipes her eyes, apologises but clearly wants to avoid me. Looking at her, sitting crumpled on the bed, I understand that I'm her worst nightmare. She doesn't want me sitting across the dinner table from her, doesn't want to know about my existence.

This is the first time I have encountered behaviour like this but not the last. Humans are pack animals and sometimes they drive the sick and wounded from the herd in order to protect the living. Those who survive often want nothing to do with those who might not. But something positive did come out of that difficult evening. Helen advises me to go to the Flemish hospital, Vrije Universiteit Brussel, known as the VUB. She tells me that they have a specialist clinic for recurrent miscarriages and that PGS might increase our chances. I note down this information. The idea of PGS makes sense to me. Surely it could increase our chances of a pregnancy that would last?

My membership of the Brussels Quaker Meeting House is confirmed. But no sooner has that happened than I start to lose whatever faith I had. I notice the moment when the cracks first appear. I am at the Quaker discussion group and the conversation is about what actually happens in a Quaker Meeting. Some people suggest that the Meeting is a space where people face up to problems in their lives and try to solve them. But for older and more experienced Quakers, the Meeting is about waiting for the presence of God – even if that presence never arrives. This latter view annoys me. Why does everything have to be so big and grand? Why does it all have to be about God?

Does it matter? I ask. I mean, if someone goes to the Meeting and as a result of an hour's silence they make a commitment to spend time with an elderly or sick relative, or if they decide to take a different approach to a colleague they find difficult, then isn't that enough? Might that not be the operation of the Spirit? Might that not be an encounter with God?

An elderly Quaker agrees that this could certainly be the case.

God is within, of course, another person says. But He could be outside as well.

I'm just not sure there is anything outside, I say. Isn't it rather dangerous for everyone always to be seeking some grand force outside themselves? Surely by focusing on the awe and mystery and otherness of God we may miss the spiritual opportunities which are right under our noses? Salvation, redemption, resurrection, epiphany – all these things exist in our daily lives. If someone who is a drug addict decides to make another attempt to give up drugs, isn't that redemption? Is that person not resurrected?

Of course, no one argues with me. They are quite happy for me to think whatever I think. But for me the moment is important. It's the beginning of the end of whatever faith I had.

And then I start to have another miscarriage. I haven't told anyone that I'm pregnant, I haven't even admitted it to myself. I have run out of reactions, of feelings. All I know is that in a few days' time we will be going on holiday and I've been look-ing forward to this holiday for months. We've rented a house called Ropehawn on a deserted stretch of coastline between St Austell and Mevagissey. Most of my family are coming to stay and also Stephen's parents and our friend Matthew from Hay-on-Wye.

I simply don't have time to have a miscarriage. Anyway a miscarriage isn't much more than a heavy period. You can get through it if you take plenty of painkillers. Dr Vermeulen has always told me that if I start to miscarry I must go to a hospi-tal because, for reasons she doesn't understand, I bleed too heavily, but I decide to ignore that.

Stephen, Thomas and I take the Eurostar to London, board the night train to Cornwall. I wake at five in the morning with mild stomach cramps and walk down the train, pull up a window. A silver expanse of water appears dotted with ghost-ly boats. Then suddenly – the sea, very close, just below the train tracks. We are travelling fast, dashing along the side of early morning breakers heading towards a tunnel opening into a cliff. I stand shivering at the open window, my hair blowing in the damp, salty wind until the train plunges into sudden blackness.

At dawn we arrive at Truro Station and pick up a hire car. I am not in too much pain. We set off for Ropehawn, Thomas in a car seat, gripping a croissant. We know that Ropehawn can't be reached by road and Thomas is discussing possible helicopter landings or pulley systems to get us to the house. The details from the letting agent instruct us to follow a track, park in a field, look out for a hand gate. The house is just below this gate and can be reached by a short track through the woods.

The track isn't short – it's long, steep and muddy, cuts its way down through a dark tunnel of brambles and trees. We struggle down gripping rucksacks and bags of food. Thomas is wobbly in his wellington boots, eyes wide, talking endlessly about smugglers, pirates, shipwrecks. Finally the track begins to level out and ahead of us is the house – tall, Victorian, painted white. And the sea, grey and churning, its long expanse stretching out far across St Austell Bay to Fowey in the far distance.

All week the weather is apocalyptic. The rain comes towards us in great sheets across the grey sea and the temperature is so low that we all wear coats and jumpers even in the house. I have come with July footwear and spend all week with mud and rain washing in at the toes of my sandals and out at the heel. I ask myself why we always go on self-catering holidays in Cornwall. Other people go to Thailand or the Caribbean. Maybe it has to do with some deep-seated English belief that pleasure isn't pleasure if it is too easily won. Flood warnings are issued all across England. Gordon Brown replaces Tony Blair as Prime Minister. We light a fire in the front room.

But despite the weather, we love the house. Mum buys a children's toy flag – a skull and crossbones – to fly from the flagpole. A cannon stands on top of a rock and Thomas wages war with imaginary pirates. A seal comes to swim outside the house each morning. Thomas catches a crab and we keep him in a bucket, christen him John.

And I swim in the sea and that's what makes the bleeding and the pain bearable. The water is so cold that I'm numb as soon as I go down into it. The coldness pressing against my chest takes my breath away but still I head out into the bay, the icy salt water splashing into my mouth. Every morning I get up and swim like this and it helps me not to think. I address the Dead Babies firmly to keep them under control. *If you want me to grieve for you, please form an orderly queue.*

XI

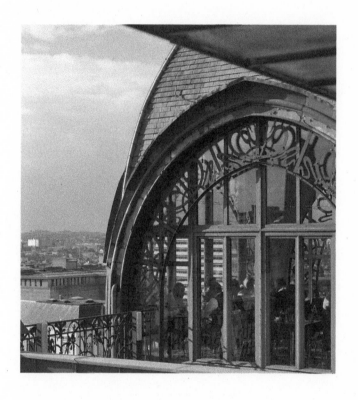

There lives more faith in honest doubt, believe me,
than in half the creeds.

Alfred, Lord Tennyson – *In Memoriam*

The sessions with Helga are working. I find a quote that seems to summarise my situation. It comes from a neurologist called Dr Paul MacLean who developed the Triune theory to explain how the brain works. This theory suggests that we all have three brains rather than one, that the modern, rational brain is built on top of two other brains, left over from earlier stages of evolution. One of these earlier brains is mammalian; the other, even older, is reptilian and is concerned only with questions of basic survival and reproduction. And so Dr MacLean says – *When a psychiatrist asks you to lie down on a couch, you're being asked to lie down with a horse and a crocodile as well.*

This quote helps me to formulate a question. Do I want to take charge of my own life? Or am I happy to let a crocodile run the show? I am determined to outwit the crocodile but at the same time I contact the VUB hospital and make an appointment, still stoking the fires of hope.

Is IVF safe? I begin to read and it soon becomes clear that no one can know about the long-term effects of IVF because the treatment is too new. But leaving aside the health issues, I soon discover that there are plenty of other reasons to be suspicious of IVF.

Firstly, despite what the media and the clinics say, it's a treatment with a low success rate. Even for a young woman with no health problems the success rate is only 20 per cent. Think of a five-sided dice. You could throw that dice many times and not get a five. Once you're over forty the success rate drops to 5 per cent or less. Think of a twenty-sided dice.

And then there's the fact that IVF is a money-making

operation. This may mean that doctors will press people to try it even though it might not be the right treatment for them. And then there are the moral objections – IVF involves generating embryos which are going to be thrown away. It leads to multiple births and an increased chance of miscarriage. And, more fundamentally, there's no shortage of babies in the world so isn't adoption a better option?

This is what I think – but I'll go ahead with the treatment anyway. My rational mind is powerless. I've given up all hope of having another baby which is alive, but IVF is the final stage in some process which must be completed and it's the completion which matters now – not the outcome. The crocodile is in control.

So Stephen and I go to the hospital recommended by Helen: the VUB. It's in Jette on the opposite side of Brussels and so the journey takes an hour – a tram down the Avenue Louise, métro to the Porte de Flandre, then a bus which winds its way out through the suburbs. It's a huge hospital, low, white and modern, spread across a patch of wasteland near to the ring road.

The doctor we see is well known in the world of infertility. People come from all over Europe and the Middle East to his clinic. So my expectations are high but, as soon as I enter his office, I know that I'm in the wrong place. I tell our story and he makes no comment at all. His eyes are fixed to his computer screen.

Yes, you should do IVF, he says.

But IVF is a treatment for people who can't get pregnant?

He tells me that PGS followed by IVF can reduce the chance of a miscarriage. But, of course, the main problem is your age, he says. You've left it too late.

I didn't leave it too late. When I had my son I was thirty-four.

But this doctor isn't interested in how we came to be in this situation. He tells me that before we start any treatment, all the tests that have been done at other hospitals will have to be redone. More sand running down through the egg timer. I should walk away but instead we agree that we'll have all the tests redone.

Our appointment with the doctor never actually ends but we are shuffled into the hands of a nurse who fills out forms.

Afterwards I say to Stephen – He didn't want us in his office.

Stephen tells me I'm paranoid. But he hasn't read about IVF so he doesn't understand how it works. IVF clinics are judged on their success rates. League tables are published online so people can decide which clinic to use. The last patient any clinic wants is a woman over forty with a history of losing babies.

You left it too late. You're too old. So how old is too old? I meet women who are getting married aged forty and are hoping to start a family. I say nothing but judge them to be hopelessly naïve. I also meet women who tell me that they aren't worried about the biological clock because of all that new technology.

These women have read a few Good News magazine articles about women of forty-eight giving birth to twins. They haven't looked into the costs – both financial and emotional – of these new technologies. They haven't read magazine articles about the women who have spent thousands of pounds, done IVF ten times, and are left with nothing. No one writes that article.

How old is too old? I always considered myself to be one of the wise virgins who tended my lamp carefully. As soon as Stephen and I got married, when I was thirty-four, I wanted us to try for a baby. I thought I was leaving myself plenty of time. But thirty-four is already too late if you have a problem, and you won't know until you try.

Of course, my opinion is far from objective. *Don't listen to her. She's cynical and bitter. Her story is so untypical that there's nothing to be learnt from it.* That's probably true but there are real questions to be answered. Twenty per cent of women are entirely infertile by the time that they're thirty-eight. This is scientific fact. Should women be trusted to find this out for themselves? I tend to think not. The modern woman is deceived but also deceives herself.

The UK government bails out Northern Rock. English expats in Brussels ask each other – what exactly is a sub-prime mortgage? Stephen and I go back and forwards to the hospital for tests. We also fill out numerous questionnaires. I look briefly at the forms that Stephen has to complete. They contain questions about premature ejaculation and erections which no one should have to answer. Wearily, Stephen writes down the details.

Of course, he says. I just have one answer to all these questions which is – No, I don't have a problem with any of these things but I soon will if you keep asking these questions.

A nurse rings from the hospital to tell me that I can't begin treatment because I have an ovarian cyst. I'm puzzled by this because I've had numerous scans over the last two years and no one has mentioned a cyst.

It's probably been caused by taking Clomid.

Right. OK. So why wasn't I warned that taking Clomid could cause this problem?

The nurse isn't interested in that conversation.

You have to go on the pill, she tells me. That might solve the problem.

So, as a woman desperate to get pregnant, I take the contraceptive pill. It's painfully clear to me that the medical profession are randomly handing out drugs with no proper understanding of the consequences. But still I do what I'm told.

I've already lost most of my faith – whatever faith I had – but in the waiting room of the IVF Clinic at the VUB in Brussels, the last drops drain away. In that place, no one looks at anyone else. Everyone is silent, ashamed, longing to be somewhere else.

But I look – at the young couples sitting there, staring at the carpet. And I see what good people they are – ordinary people, with scrubbed-clean faces and tidy clothes and innocent eyes. And all these people want is a baby. They don't want to win the lottery, or travel the world, or be awarded an Oscar. They just want a baby – a desire that is well within the realms of what they can reasonably expect.

But these people have waited and waited. And they've done the tests, and answered the intrusive questions, and the women have had endless probes stuck up them, and the men have masturbated into tubes. And now their marriages are stretched to breaking point, and they don't understand. Why? Why? For most of them there is no explanation and there never will be.

They are the barren. That's a word that isn't used any more because it sounds so cruel – but it is deadly accurate. The barren. The people whose love has failed to spark new life. Most of these people are in a situation much worse than mine. I have a living child, and a dead child, a collection of miscarried foetuses. I get pregnant. For many of these people, it's just endless waiting and nothing and nothing and nothing.

There is no loving and good God, there can't be. Why did I ever think there was? Only because I had it banged into me from childhood. How could I have been so deceived? There are great forces out there, I know that, but those forces are utterly indifferent to human need, to human suffering.

Losing my faith isn't a painful process. Instead it's a huge relief. I put it down as one drops a heavy and awkward bag. A bag that has stretched my arm out of its socket, a bag whose sharp edges have scratched against my legs. A bag that simply never fitted properly anywhere. Always the wrong size and the wrong shape, it wouldn't go under the bed or into any cupboard.

So finally I just leave it on the side of the road, and walk on weightless and smiling. I no longer need to search for meanings or for lessons. I no longer need to turn suffering to account, to bring good out of evil. I don't need to rewrite the story so that it has a positive ending. Nietzsche said – *To live is to suffer, to survive is to find some meaning in suffering.* But personally I suspect that the need to find meaning is an unnecessary burden laid at the door of the bereaved.

Instead I can cheerfully give way to despair – a state that I soon discover to be much underestimated. The great virtue of despair is that you know where you stand with it. You expect absolutely nothing so you can't be disappointed. And once you have it – despair, this pearl of great value – then everything else clears away. Whatever small goodness you find is infinitely special. You stop complaining about why the world is not as you want it to be, as you'd been told it would be. As R. S. Thomas says – *Life is struggle, nothing more.*

Joslin rings and wails down the telephone. I go around to her house.

I need your help, she says. But you're the last person I should ask for help. I'm so sorry. But I've just got to tell you straight out.

But I already know.

You're pregnant?

Yes. And I didn't want to get pregnant. I'm just not in a situation where I should have another child. And he doesn't want another.

I could be furious with her but, given how confused I am about my own fertility, I can hardly criticise. I've been in this situation many times before. Women who are well into their thirties who become pregnant 'by accident' despite the fact that they've been using contraception successfully for the last fifteen years.

Some part of you wanted this, I say.

Yes. I suppose so. But I didn't.

If Joslin were another woman, I would simply walk out, suggest that she should go somewhere else for help. But Joslin has looked after me over the last few months, she's tried to understand and she knows how difficult this is for me. And she is incredibly strong, she's already rallying, wiping her eyes, beginning to laugh. She's bending her mind to this new reality and she'll soon succeed in deciding that this is all for the best after all. She has no other choice. She takes me into the kitchen, makes tea.

Isn't this a bloody awful, unfair world? There's you desperate for a baby. And I don't want one and now I'm going to have one.

No one can ever really be sad about a baby coming into the world, can they? I say.

Two months later the cyst disappears and Stephen and I go to meet the doctor at the VUB again so that he can give us the results of all the tests. Stephen is worried about this appointment because, for the first time, he's being tested as well as me. Maybe it's going to turn out that he has a problem? He's a modern man but still this would be difficult for him. It's easier for both of us if I'm the one with the problem.

The doctor goes through the tests results, looks at Stephen.

You have a sperm count of five million.

Stephen sits up straighter, squares his shoulders.

Which is normal, the doctor says.

Stephen deflates although he's still relieved that none of this seems to be to do with him. The results of all my tests also reveal nothing.

You can start IVF. Go to the desk. They'll give you an appointment with a counsellor.

I assume that a person with the title counsellor has some sort of advisory role but the woman we meet only talks about drugs. I tell her that I'm still unclear whether this is the right decision for us. She isn't interested. The waiting list is long, we are lucky we can start so soon. She explains that I will need to give myself daily injections.

I can't do that.

Oh. Well, you could come to the hospital.

It takes me an hour to get here.

It soon becomes clear that I've got no choice about the injections. The counsellor explains that this isn't an injection that involves veins. That's a relief but still I lie awake in the night worrying about how I will stick a needle in myself – particularly as Stephen is going to be away on a business trip at the time when I need to start.

I go to the pharmacy in the basement of the hospital to be given the drugs. I'm handed a bulging carrier bag – and this is only the start of what will be needed. The whole process is mysterious and unpredictable. It feels like *Mission: Impossible*. I receive cryptic phone calls from the hospital every day telling me what to do. But the instructions aren't – *Leave the money in an unmarked envelope in the phone box at the corner of the street.* Instead I'm told to go to the hospital for this test, or that, or to stop taking this drug and start taking that.

The day of the first injection arrives. As ever, it turns out I've been worrying about the wrong thing. Breaking open the little glass phials which contain the medication and mixing it turns out to be the complicated part. Once I've done that I'm ready to go. The injection has to be done at a certain time and I can't delay.

Downstairs the doorbell rings. I hear Big Alice, who is downstairs, open the front door and then I hear a piercing wail. From the conversation it's clear that Thomas has been in the park with friends and has got sand in his eyes. I sit down and stick the needle into the lower part of my stomach. Then I run downstairs to look after Thomas and feel half grateful to him for his eye problem.

I can't predict anything. The appointments are always at anti-social hours. I soon get quite confident with the needle. I learn to do it fast, hard with a smooth flick of the wrist, oddly like playing darts. My arms are sore from all the blood tests. Surely they've taken all the blood that I have by now? I also have to go for endless scans.

Wait until your number comes up and then enter a cubicle. Remove the lower half of your clothing. Wait for a light to go on, open the door at the other end of the cubicle and enter a room dominated by stirrups. Medical staff have masks over their faces. The lights are low. You climb onto a high bed and your feet are locked into place. Then they stick a probe into your vagina.

Everyone accepts that such procedures are sometimes necessary. But when they've done this to you four times in a week it does begin to feel like rape. If I felt like having any sense of humour, then the scans would make me laugh because the probe looks just like a penis and they cover it with a plastic thing that looks exactly like a condom. But I'm well past the possibility of comedy.

Occasionally the person doing the scan tries to engage me in conversation – or in what passes for conversation in this hospital. They make comments on how the process is progressing. They even invite me to look on the screen. They say mysterious things like – you have four follicles. Is that good or bad? I'm not even interested in finding out. I fix them with a nasty stare that makes clear that they should leave me out of this.

Sometimes – when Thomas is at nursery – I get in the car and drive to the car park at Altitude Cent. Brussels is largely a flat city but from this minor peak there is a view – across miles of blocks of flats, railway lines, office buildings. The sun glistens on the dome of the Palais de Justice, the spire of the Hôtel de Ville in the Grand Place. I sit in the car and scream – and scream and scream. Then I smash my fists up and down on the steering wheel, scream, cry, scream again.

Afterwards I go home and take a solid metal cooking pot from the cupboard and, kneeling down, smash it onto the tiles again and again, as hard as I can. I wait for the tiles to crack or the pan to buckle, but material things – pans and tiles – are far more resilient than the human heart.

I decide that since my body is being poisoned by the medical profession, then I have to look after myself in every other way possible. I become obsessed by eating healthy food, go to endless yoga classes. Another mysterious call comes telling me that it's time to go to the hospital for the egg collection. This will involve a day in the hospital, an anaesthetic, an operating theatre, plenty more drugs. Stephen goes to the hospital with me that day so that he can masturbate into a test tube. The nurse says – Perhaps you would like to go into the cubicle with your husband?

Stephen and I stare at her in confusion.

Some couples like to do that, she says. To join together in this intimacy.

Stephen and I start to laugh and we can't stop. Is this woman seriously suggesting that this process has got something to do with pleasure? Do they really think that Stephen and I are going to have a romantic moment in a hospital cubicle with a plastic curtain for a door? The two of us rediscovering our love for each other as I give him a hand job and we both aim for the tube?

Over the next two days the hospital tries to fertilise the eggs. My eggs meeting Stephen's sperm somewhere in a test tube in Jette. This is what our marriage has come to now. I am exhausted and wander through the city aimlessly. Eventually I stop at the Musical Instrument Museum and take the lift up to the café – an eyrie of intricate Art Nouveau ironwork high above the city. I'm sitting there drinking a herb tea and staring out over the grey haze of the city when a call comes telling me that tomorrow I need to go to the hospital for the transfer. I'm told that before the transfer I will have an appointment with a geneticist.

The next day I find myself lying on an operating trolley inadequately wrapped in a green sheet. A woman comes in wearing a mask and tells me that they were only able to harvest three eggs and only two developed and so they will implant these. This is the appointment with the geneticist.

But what about the PGS?

Oh, we can't do that for you. You don't have enough eggs.

But that's the whole reason I'm here.

Yes, but you don't have enough eggs.

OK – so how many women over the age of forty don't have enough eggs?

Oh, most of them.

So then why was I offered a treatment that was unlikely to work for me?

It's clear that this geneticist didn't even know that we'd been expecting PGS. A minor administrative error. But for us the last hope has gone. I am reminded of a woman on an internet message board who described IVF as an expensive way of letting people down gently. I'm wheeled in for the transfer. Nurses talk over me in Flemish as they work, laughing and nudging each other.

Oh dear, they say. It seems that one of the embryos might have got lost. Maybe it got dropped on the floor.

But then they check again. No problem. Found it.

After the treatment, I lie in a hospital bed. Outside I can see nothing except a patch of white sky. I'm numb with drugs but inside I ache, like bad period pain. I hate myself for doing this and I hate this place. In this world, a child dies every ten seconds due to lack of clean drinking water and yet here am I, in this large new specialist hospital unit, totally dedicated to filling women up with drugs to produce babies. The whole thing stinks and yet I'm part of it.

And then some strange shift takes place in my mind and I wake up and I'm somewhere up above the hospital bed looking down at myself. And there I am: a forty-two-year-old woman, lying in a hospital bed. A woman who is perfectly healthy but who has chosen to make herself ill in the pursuit of something she can't have. A clear message had been sent to me – you will not have another baby who is alive. And yet I have argued and argued with that. And this now is the result. I have turned into a person that I do not like.

Who was I before this happened to me? I know the answer immediately. It comes to me in an image of my younger self. There I am – on a boat, or a ferry, travelling somewhere. I don't know where. When I was young I was always travelling somewhere, usually with no map and no money. Egypt, Turkey, Indonesia, Thailand, China, South America. The train from Brussels to Beijing.

Where is that imagined boat? Possibly on its way to the Aeolian Isles, or crossing from Java to Bali. The sun is hot and the wind brisk. I'm out on deck, standing beside white painted railings, looking out to sea. I'm wearing shorts and a blue cotton jumper with a striped blue and white T-shirt underneath. This is the person I used to be.

And suddenly I decide. I'm not going to see any more doctors. I'm not going to be a pathetic woman, crying in a hospital bed. Instead I'm going to find my way back to that other self who stands on the deck of the ferry, her hair blown back from her face. A woman who is travelling without fear to a destination unknown.

The IVF fails. A nurse phones to give me this news. The phone call lasts for less than a minute. She advises me not to make an appointment to see a doctor. The doctors prefer not to see you for a few weeks, she says, because people do tend to get rather emotional.

XII

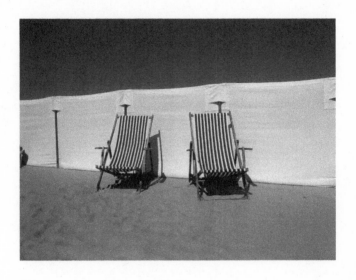

It's not what happens to you, but how
you react to it that matters.

Epictetus

Then – I find it hard to write this, hard to believe it – we do IVF again. Even now I can't work out how this happened. I would like to blame it on the hospital but it isn't that simple. Initially we go back to see the doctor at the VUB just to ask for advice. We should be confronting him about the fact that he gave us information that was misleading but neither of us has the energy for that conversation.

Stephen is determined that we should understand all the possible choices. I already know there are no choices. What we need is for someone to shoot us in the foot. Of course, we should do it ourselves but for months now we've been passing the gun back and forwards between us, failing to take aim. The best we can hope for is that someone with a good nerve and a steady aim will do the job for us. But this doctor is not the man for the job. He's better at computer screens.

So is there any point in us doing IVF again? Stephen asks.

The doctor is impatient. Oh, I really can't make that decision for you.

Power without responsibility.

The appointment never comes to any definite end, no conclusion is reached, but instead we're edged out of the door, handed over to nurses. These people handle me as though I'm full of poisonous liquid that might spill and burn. Perhaps the rage is beginning to show on my skin like a red and itching rash.

We begin to discuss dates with the counsellor. It's early April and we leave Brussels in the summer. There's a waiting list and we can't be accommodated. I hear the words and know that we're being offered a way out. The hills are ahead of us, run towards them, a clean break. Stephen and I look at each other. If we accept what she's saying then we're at the end of hope.

I lose my nerve, swerve back through the prison gates.

You must find a date. You must.

She prevaricates.

I'm not leaving this office until you sort out a date.

I watch myself from a distance, a hideous lump of barnacled rage. I can't believe what I'm doing. We know that the chances of IVF working are 5 per cent or less, we know that the PGS can't work for us. We know that even if I get pregnant the chances of a miscarriage are at least 60 per cent. And yet here I am, blindly fighting for an invasive and unpleasant treatment that I don't want. But still this seems easier than the howling black abyss that is the other option.

Nurses are hovering, looking nervous. Everyone – Stephen included – is moving carefully now because the poisonous liquid is right at the brim and the slightest wrong move may spread it, burning, everywhere. The counsellor consults her papers nervously. Something can be arranged, a phone call is made, and it is agreed that in two months we'll start on a new cycle of treatment.

Joslin calls me to tell me that she went for a three month scan and the doctors found no heartbeat. I did know, she says. I did feel something was wrong.

I'm sorry. I'm so sorry.

I'm all right. But can you tell me how it works, what I have to do?

I explain to her that she will have a choice between going into hospital and staying at home, taking pills. She says immediately she'll stay at home. She wants to see the baby – if there is anything to see – and she wants to have a funeral. She has decided to call the baby Nancy Grace.

I hate bloody earth-mother, soul-enhancing Joslin. No

doubt she'll organise a beautiful ceremony and turn the whole experience into something positive and meaningful. And she'll create some fantastic artwork expressing all that she feels about the loss of this baby. Why am I not like that?

I always just want the anaesthetic, I say. Loads of drugs and that's it.

Three days later she calls again. The baby has gone – and now her marriage as well. Both in the same week. We often talk about our lives like a game of poker and now she says – I'll see your four Dead Babies and raise you divorce and miscarriage in the same week. But behind the black humour, she is shattered.

I just woke up the morning after the miscarriage, she says. And I had to know. So I just went to see her – the woman. Said – Have you been sleeping with my husband? She admitted she has. And he promised me, he absolutely promised me, it wasn't true. So now it's finished because I don't trust anything he says.

I look at her. She's always been a person who exists without the usual means of support. She's an only child and, although she has parents, they are so unreasonable that she never sees them. Now she is alone with two children and the pain of betrayal. She can cope with what he's done to her but not what he's doing to his children. But still she's controlled, strong, certain.

I'll move back to England, she says. Find a job teaching fine art.

I ask her about the miscarriage. Sure enough, just the day before, when she still had a marriage, she organised a funeral for Nancy Grace.

She's buried in the garden, Joslin says. And the children

painted pictures for her and they made a special tea, planted
flowers.

Lovely, I say.

You big liar, Joslin says. You don't think that at all.

No. I do. It's just the details. It seems a bit gross.

Well, yes. It was, Joslin says. To be honest. I mean, I put her
– well, what I thought was her – in a Tupperware pot but then
I didn't know what to do. And so finally I put her in the fridge
but I did worry a bit, you know, in case, someone was looking
in the fridge. You know.

Looking for what?

Well, I don't know. Tomato salsa?

Suddenly we're both convulsed with laughter. Joslin col-
lapses against the kitchen units, my hand bangs up and down
on the table. We shake and shudder, wipe up tears. Joslin
slides down to the floor and I go and get a cushion for her,
place it under her head, sit beside her. There's a sense of relief
in all this. She's put up with the rumours, the lying, too long.

She doesn't want to finish up in a wrangle with him. People
at the Meeting House have offered to help with mediation,
negotiation. She won't give in to bitterness and hatred. I have
a great respect for the Quakers and their skills in negotiation,
peacemaking. But I've seen many ugly divorces – my parents'
included. And I know the kind of man her husband is.

Lovely, I say. But I'd hire a good lawyer and take him for
every penny.

Joslin isn't listening. She's still sure that something can be
salvaged. She makes a plan, we both of us make plans. Going
back to the UK, new lives, possibilities. Joslin has four weeks
of school holidays ahead of her and nothing particular to do,
other than look after the children. I have two months until I
have to start IVF again. Joslin says she can't stay in the house

in Brussels. So she'll go on a trip around the UK, taking the children with her, going to visit old friends.

It'll work out fine, the children can sleep in the car, or we can camp.

New lives. Travel. Moving on. I can't wait two months, I need to go somewhere now. I need to become the young woman on the boat. Also, as I'm only ever going to have one child, I need to find a positive story to tell about that. It soon occurs to me that the two objectives fit neatly together. The truth is – I force myself to admit it – that the fact that Laura died means that I can travel more easily. With two children you're a sitting duck, you can only wait until the bullet finds you. If you have one child, you can pick it up and run.

Thomas, do you want to go to Venice?

OK. Can we go on the tram? Do they have ice cream?

Ice cream – certainly.

I book the night train to Venice for Thomas and me. Stephen is away on a business trip to America so he can't come with us. I also book rooms in the Hôtel Des Bains on the Lido. I've always wanted to stay in this hotel because it's where Thomas Mann wrote *Death in Venice*. I borrow a wheelie suitcase from a friend and plan carefully so that everything will fit in that one bag.

I'm not deceiving myself about this. I've done enough of the grief business to know that this is one of those strange bursts of energy that comes with loss. But I've also learnt that when this nervous euphoria comes you should ride the wave for all it's worth, knowing that soon enough it will come crashing down on top of you and you'll be washed back down to the depths.

Thomas and I set out for the Gare du Midi, take the fast train to Paris, pull our one bag behind us through the métro and arrive at Paris Bercy. The next morning we come out of the Venice Central station onto the Grand Canal and gasp. The sun is bright and the whole of Venice glitters before us. We stand up in the back of the water taxi, speechless.

When booking the Hôtel Des Bains, I'd failed to realise that the hotel is always closed for the winter months. So we arrive on the day when it opens for the summer, the first and only guests. Dated and stately, the hotel is a 1920s palace of white stucco, surrounded by acres of parkland, with its own private beach.

Inside, a museum of faded splendour awaits – a forest of white marble pillars, expanses of creaking parquet, warped wooden shutters, heavy mahogany furniture with gilt twiddles. Everything is marble, crystal, wood. Everything tarnished and worn. The ghosts of Scott and Zelda Fitzgerald, Noël Coward, dance the Charleston on the terraces.

Now Thomas and I are alone in these endless corridors, waited on by scores of bored young men in full livery who challenge Thomas to games of cards and bring him far too much ice cream. We go straight down to the beach and, as the sun is out, Thomas strips off and plays in the sand. Later, we take the boat back to St Mark's and see the basilica, stand on a bridge and watch the gondoliers crowded into a narrow canal below. I comment on the splendour of the scene.

Thomas groans – Beauty, beauty, beauty. That's all you talk about.

When we get back to the hotel, a storm suddenly blows in. Thunder snaps, sudden gusts of rain batter on the terrace awnings. Footmen hurry to close wildly swinging shutters. As the light falls, Thomas and I play cricket with a loo brush and a rolled-up pair of socks in the empty corridors, our game illuminated by flashes of lightening which spill across the parquet.

The next morning we hire a four-wheeled bicycle and pedal all around the Lido. The bicycle is shielded from the sun by a canvas roof. Thomas has to stand up to pedal. Once we get stuck on a steep bridge but cheerful Italians crowd behind us and push us up to the ridge, then cheer as we sail away down the other side.

In the afternoon, we turn our bike off the beach front and head over to the other side of the island. Taking a random turn we finish up on the banks of the lagoon looking out over Venice itself. We decide to stop here as we need a break and there's a bench and shady trees on the bank.

It's a nothing kind of place – just a No Through Road at the end of a line of suburban villas. And yet we stay there for an hour or more. I sit on the banks of the lagoon staring out at the city and watching boats pass by. Thomas begins an elaborate game of gangster which involves climbing all over the four-wheeled bike. Occasionally people pass by walking dogs.

I know that I'll remember this particular nondescript little spot long after the more dramatic moments of the trip have faded. It's always like that. Always the lay-by one remembers, or the ford where one stopped to paddle, or the track which one walked down to have a pee.

These are the places that remain. Probably because one comes at them with no expectation or desire and so one enjoys them exactly as they are. Whereas the dramatic sights are loaded with one hundred preconceived ideas and so disappoint, are easily forgotten. At the end of this nondescript No Through Road, I want for nothing.

On our last day, as we're heading back to the station, we stop to feed the pigeons in St Mark's Square. For Thomas this is the highlight of the trip. I take photographs of him with two pigeons on each arm, one on his head. Then we have tea in Florian's and it's like sitting inside a jewellery box. A waiter brings a gold tasselled cushion for Thomas to sit on. A string quartet is playing outside and we can see out onto the square – elegant, crumbling, dirty.

Thomas rolls his eyes and says – I could eat sixty cakes like this.

Everyone in the room is laughing at him and he knows it. I watch him and suddenly it's like falling completely and absolutely in love. That upside down, vertigo feeling. All the air gone from my lungs.

Exhausted by Venice, we sleep well on the journey back and fail to realise that the train has arrived in Paris. We're woken by an irate guard banging on our door telling us that we have one minute to vacate the train. And so we drag our bag down the platform, laughing, and travel all the way back to Brussels still wearing our pyjamas. What a relief it is to live again.

But back in Brussels the IVF starts – and I scream often. Not just in the car, on my own, parked up at Altitude Cent, but in the street, the hospital. I go for a blood test and am told that I need different drugs. These drugs won't be available until tomorrow so I will have to come back to the hospital again.

Do you realise that it takes me an hour to get to this hospital?

Oh – where do you live?

Ixelles.

It doesn't take an hour to get from Ixelles to here.

I start screaming. Fuck, fuck, fuck, fuck, fuck. I go on and on. The nurse stands watching me petulantly.

It's not my fault.

I didn't fucking well say it was.

Fuck, fuck, fuck. She pushes me out of the room into the corridor, shuts the door on me. I look up to find a row of people staring at me. I wonder if anyone will get up and offer me assistance but they stare at the floor, fumble with the clasp of a handbag, ease the collar of a shirt. They have been schooled in the etiquette of this hospital. Do not meet anyone's eye, do not talk to other patients.

I go to the loos and scream, kick the wall hard. I'm wearing boots with black rubber soles and they leave marks on the pristine walls. I'm glad about this. My toe aches from all the kicking. Later I'll find that I've broken one of my nails. Finally I give up and go down to the foyer, intending to catch a bus home.

It's seven o'clock by now and the foyer is deserted, the reception desk shut up. The rain is coming down like a shower and the bus stop is ten minutes' walk. I sit down to wait, hoping the rain might ease, ring my mum and my sister. Usually I try not to bother them as they've got enough troubles of their own.

My sister says – Fantastic. Well done. You should do that a lot more often.

I'm grateful to her and even start laughing as I describe the scene, but in truth I'm ashamed of myself. Until two years ago I was always polite and reasonable. Perhaps that's part of the problem. Perhaps I've been storing all this up for the last forty-two years and the dam has finally burst. But I find it hard to accept this new version of myself. I remember all the stories I've heard of those people who've got cancer for the third time and they're still smiling at the hospital staff and being tremendously courageous and pleasant. It turns out that I'm not that kind of person.

Over the next few days my mood changes, my mind eases. We'll be leaving Brussels in a few months now, so I am packing up the house. This should be a dismal process but I feel dangerously well. I go for the egg collection and I am purposefully charming to everyone in the hospital. This is not Zimbabwe or the Horn of Africa, it's a middle-class English tragedy. The nurses in the hospital are almost pleasant to me. I make a note to myself to make more effort to remember that what you give out in life is what you get back.

Joslin is packing as well, preparing for her trip around the UK and also for leaving Brussels permanently. When my friend Matthew comes to stay, she likes him immediately, writes Hay-on-Wye into her plans, looks happier than she has done in weeks. We speak on the phone in the evening, comparing notes. In reality, our situations are quite different. Stephen and I are going together to Mount Vernon, in Gloucestershire, a house we own. Joslin is alone with two children and she has no idea where she'll go. Predictably it's fast becoming clear that her ex-husband isn't going to give her a penny if he can avoid it.

I feel like a big red balloon, sailing through the sky, full of hope and promise, cheerfully waving in the wind. But it will only take one thorn and the balloon will be gone. Nothing left but a small and twisted piece of rubber. In two days it will be the third anniversary of Laura's death. In five days we get the results of the IVF. Foolishly, foolishly I'm beginning to think that it might have worked.

Stephen and I decide that we'll go to the coast together on Laura's anniversary. We take the train to Ostend, passing through fields that are low, green and secret. Huge white cows graze below lines of poplars that stretch across the landscape, edging canals which brim full of glassy water. We pass low red farms, bland back gardens with trampolines, paddling pools, deckchairs.

From Ostend we pick up the tram that runs the entire length of the twenty-three miles of the Belgian coast. We get off at a small town which I have visited often before called La Coq in French, De Haan in Flemish. It's a curious place. The houses are mainly half-timbered – black and white like those on a sedate 1930s housing estate in England. The tram stop – and in fact the whole place – has a Toy Town feeling to it. Tidy, quaint, suburban. It feels colonial, appears to have been imported from somewhere else.

Couples cut into *steak-frites* in the steamed-up windows of the restaurants along the seafront. Stephen and I have brought books with us, and we hire blue-and-white-striped deckchairs, tuck them in under a windbreak, sit and read. Briefly the tugging wind drops and the sun comes out. My eyes roam the gables of the seafront, move out to the blurred grey horizon. Everything is just as it should be.

But by the time we get home, I've discovered that I'm bleeding so I can't be pregnant. This is hardly surprising but the timing is outrageous. There are 365 days in a year and we have to get this news at this time. We won't do IVF again and so that's it – the end.

XIII

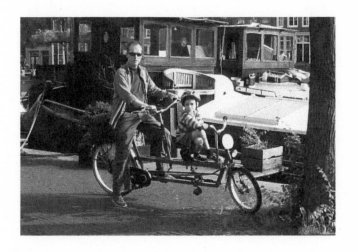

God is a comedian playing to an audience
that is too afraid to laugh.

Voltaire

Hindsight. I need it like a lung patient needs oxygen. I'm struggling to keep a grip on the rage. In memoirs the case for the defence is never heard. But I now need to construct that case, if only to calm myself. The IVF experience did nothing except make a bad situation worse. But who can I blame for this? Finally, only myself. We were not victims, we were volunteers.

And of course, I'd be telling a very different story if the IVF had worked. I know plenty of people for whom it has worked, people who owe their children to it. For those people the humiliation and pain, the emotional turmoil, have largely been wiped from their memories because they've won the ultimate prize – a live baby.

The truth is that Stephen and I should never have embarked on IVF because I wasn't in a mental state where I could cope. But given the international reputation of the VUB, why did no one there see what was happening? The truth is that people with infertility issues are often gullible, desperate and mad. They need protecting from themselves. I can say that because I was one of those people. Who protects such people? Who tells them the truth? Who has the courage to kill their hope?

Move. Just keep moving. I arrange for us all to go to Amsterdam for the weekend. As soon as we arrive at our hotel on the Prinsengracht Canal, I'm fired with an energy that buzzes like an electric shock. I'm in love with the tall, red-brick gabled houses, the carless streets, the eccentric shops with their flower-power fabrics and 70s kitsch. This city is as watery as Venice but satisfyingly dour, eccentric, unpretentious.

As soon as we get back home, I book for us to go again in two weeks' time, but this time we're staying on a houseboat. Stephen doesn't argue. Is he just humouring me? Or does he too need to keep moving?

This time we're better organised and hire bikes. I ride one bike and Stephen and Thomas share a tandem. Thomas is at the front and has a steering wheel which isn't connected to anything but he thinks he's navigating our route through the city.

We go to the paddling pool in the Vondelpark, the zoo, we pedal for miles in search of a windmill. This is Holland. We must find a windmill. Finally we find one but it's closed. Thomas doesn't mind. At least he's seen the outside of a windmill. Do not stop. Keep on pedalling.

Later we go out on a boat across the grey, choppy water which smells of drains, and then finally head back to the houseboat and cook ourselves supper and eat up on deck while the city spins past us. I don't want to go back home to the packing, the pain, the loneliness.

A few days later I'm out with Stephen and we finish up in a trendy bar in the next street to our house. It is all stainless steel and red leather chairs like an American diner. Tubes of fluorescent light glitter behind the bar and the waitresses have six-inch heels, bare midriffs.

I finish up in conversation with a woman I vaguely know. She wears a small, tight black dress with a belt as thin as a ribbon. Her dark hair is cut short, her mascara carefully applied so that each eyelash remains separate. Her nails are painted with a flawless layer of translucent glaze. We've both had a little too much to drink and have to shout above the pulse of the music.

This woman is thirty-eight and she's been wanting a child for some years. But her partner of ten years feels the time isn't right. She's worried that he might be having an affair, concerned that the relationship isn't right for her anyway. She doesn't want to leave him but equally she doesn't want a life without children.

I think of all the stories I've read on infertility websites. All those women in their early forties who've patiently waited for the right time, only to be dumped for someone younger. Women who are now discovering the reality of all that impressive new technology.

If I were you, I say, I'd just get pregnant and claim it was an accident.

Those mascara eyes open wide. Her head goes back, her earrings swing.

That's appalling.

Yes, I know. Ten years ago I'd have thought the same.

No, she says. No. I couldn't trap a man like that.

Yes. But you may be facing a choice. Do you want to be forty-five and divorced with two children? Or do you want to be forty-five and divorced with no children? I'd suggest the former.

You're very cynical, she says.

Yes, I am. But I've seen too many women miss their chance.

I look at her – shiny, unstained. Living in a child-free, office-working world. A world of manicures and definite moral judgements. I wish I were her. I wish I didn't know what I know. She shrugs, tosses her head, waves a dove-like hand in a gesture that suggests dismissal. She doesn't like me and she doesn't like my advice. I don't like me much either.

It's only a month now until we leave Brussels, the city that has been Stephen's home for over twenty years and mine for sixteen. I spend every day packing up the house. I find bags lying under the dining room table that we packed to go on some outing two years ago and have been there ever since.

For years I have believed so strongly in taking possession of the past as a means of understanding the present, shaping the future. Now all I want is to forget. I want to get rid of everything, everything. Many of the things I take to the junk market are perfectly good and might even have been useful, but I just don't want to see them again in England. I want to start again.

It's the end of July now and everything is closing down, everyone is leaving, heading down to the south. We don't have a leaving party, I don't say goodbye to anyone. On the final Sunday, I'm intending to go to the Meeting House to say farewell to all the people there who have looked after me with such love over the last three years, but then I decide not to go.

I keep telling myself that it doesn't matter that we're leaving. The life that we used to have here doesn't exist any more so why stay? The whole place is stained by the events of the last three years. Every restaurant we pass is a place where we went when I was pregnant, every tram line leads to one hospital or another, every street corner is the scene of a strained and difficult conversation. Time for us to go.

Four days until we leave this city. I'm packing now late into the night. Stephen is busy at work and says – Don't worry. It'll get done somehow. But it won't get done unless I do it. The walls of the house are stripped bare, suitcases and cardboard boxes block the corridors and doorways. Whole swathes of my past have been carted away to the charity shop, and loads more are by the door, ready to go.

And Laura's rose bush in the garden? I take advice and find that this isn't the right time of year to move it. Stephen speaks to the people who are buying the house and asks if we can come back to take the bush later and they agree to this. But when will we ever manage to come back? Do the airlines or Eurostar allow passengers to travel with an uprooted rose bush?

The moment comes when I need to take Thomas's bike to the junk market and my nerve fails me. Thomas has outgrown the bike and it was always horrid anyway. My mother got it from a dump. It's black and orange – a combination of colours I particularly dislike. The word Foxy is painted on the crossbar.

Last summer I spent hours with Thomas and Foxy, teaching him to ride without stabilisers. We've done all the parks in Brussels on that bike and he's ridden it all around my mum's farm as well. And so now I just can't put Foxy in the back of the car and take him to the junk market.

So I give up for a while, sit out on the terrace, amidst piles of garden implements, and drink tea. It's funny the odd things which tug at the heart strings, the bits of the past which refuse to be cut adrift. Strangely it isn't the people we know here that I'll miss but odd, insignificant things. The people at the florists in the square who we say good morning to every day. And our elderly neighbours.

Immaculately dressed, they walk out together, hand in hand. He has a cloud of white hair, she has a smile which lights up the whole street. They talk to us about the war, express their gratitude for the part England played in the Allied victory. Together they are a reminder of some other life that existed in this city, before the European Union arrived and the Moroccan Sans Papiers. Marooned here now they tend their garden, disappear at the weekends down to their country house in Namur. I will die of this leaving. It is one loss too many.

The plan is that we will leave now, at the end of July, and then I'll come back to the house one more time in September, before the packers arrive, to see everything loaded up. But the day of departure comes and we're late for the ferry. The things we'll need for the next six weeks are pushed into the car hurriedly. I don't even have time to walk through the rooms of the house to say goodbye. I tell myself that this doesn't matter because I'll be back in September.

Briefly I stand at the French windows, stare out down the long, narrow walled garden with the arch at the end, the espaliered trees behind, the roof of the convent beyond. But Stephen and Thomas are calling me so I have to go.

And so we set out, our Peugeot 106 groaning under the weight of luggage, rolling down the Avenue Louise, past the Porte de Flandre and the Basilique. On to the road which will lead out through those miles of flat land, spreading out towards Calais, the coast, the sea.

In September, plans change. I never go back to that house.

XIV

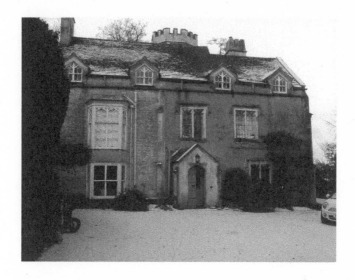

We have to pretend.
If we don't pretend, we are lost.

Stendhal

Our house in England – Mount Vernon – is a fantasy house. Built of Cotswold stone, perched on a ledge above the town of Stroud, it is the last house on the Cotswold escarpment, marking the point where the land drops away to the Severn Vale. Hidden among trees, it has a tower and battlements, arched windows with delicate tracery, as fine and frothy as lace. A gothic folly, a miniature fort, it is both frivolous and gloomy, like an abandoned wedding cake.

On a winter's evening, it becomes the villain's castle in a Hammer Horror film, with ragged rooks screaming around the tower. Ghosts appear at the gothic windows, their skirts rustle on the many stairs. A mad woman is shut up in the tower. But on a honey-coloured summer's day, it's a fairy-tale palace and has that castaway look of houses beside the sea.

In reality, Mount Vernon is nowhere near the sea, but in the evenings we can walk up through the woods to the gate which leads onto Rodborough Common and, if we climb on up from there, onto the blustery roof of the hills, we can see a distant ribbon of silver glinting through the landscape below. This is the River Severn, growing in force and width as it slides out towards the Bristol Channel. Standing there, I feel myself washed out to Portishead, Clevedon, Weston-super-Mare, the open sea.

Thomas and I arrive at Mount Vernon in August 2008 with only our suitcases and a blow-up air bed. The grass on the lawn is long, trees press in close, creepers twist across the windows. The house smells of damp plaster and garden earth. The wallpaper is pale green and peeling. Rags are tied around dripping taps in distant sculleries. The floors are bare wood, speckled with nails, where the carpets have been pulled up.

It's evening and Thomas and I walk through the shadowy rooms, sure we've been here before. The house is built on eight interlocking floors so it is easy to get lost. Turning suddenly, we expect to find a stranger's face in a lone gilt mirror left hanging on a landing, but discover only our own furtive eyes. Thomas goes to an arched stone window, calls to me urgently. Through the dusty glass we see deer grazing on the lawn. They look up and see us, stare imperiously. This is their world and we have invaded it.

We blow up the air bed, spread out our sleeping bags, moving quietly so as not to disturb the deer, the hovering ghosts. As I head down through the blunt echoes of the house, past the grey sparkle of evening windows, I notice Thomas following behind me.

Are you frightened?

Mummy, I didn't want to say – but I am frightened.

So I grip his hot little hand in mine. This should be a moment of excitement and it is. But behind the excitement is fear. We bought this house at a time when we were different people. We had some crazy plan about a commune, or at the very least hordes of friends coming to stay. But the friends don't exist any more. We should sell the house and get something more practical but we won't do that. We owe Mount Vernon something. We are in this together now.

But the whole place needs restoring. The work will take years. On the top floor is the room that, when we bought the house, I earmarked for the daughter I hoped to have. Laura's room. A small room with sloping ceilings, a tiny pointed window and a chipboard floor. I'm still going to make it into a little girl's room even though there's no little girl to live in it. After Thomas is settled on the air bed, I stand at the window, trying out my new mobile phone. Every time I send a text the phone changes my name from Alice to Alive.

At Mount Vernon there are magpies everywhere – single magpies. How does the magpie species continue given that they never meet? Separate, sinister, they squat along the top lane and swoop away over the Common. Ragged and hopping, with tiny shallow eyes, sharp beaks and a shiny blue gleam to their grubby piebald feathers, they dance in trees on our drive and, in the early morning, stretch worms from the lawn. I'm not superstitious – or I never used to be. But I'm haunted by them. Haven't we had our share of bad luck?

When I left England in my late twenties I was determined I would never return. But now Thomas is going to the neighbouring school to the one I myself attended. As I drive him there I say to myself – *Remind me again, what am I doing back here?* But what I need now is familiarity. I can't be an adventurer or a traveller any more. And overall, I'm glad that Thomas is going to a school that I understand. Becoming a parent makes you conventional. You want your child to have the same childhood as you, even though it did you no good.

Joslin comes to stay, leaving the children with her mother-in-law. She is still living in Brussels but plans to move to England soon. She needs to rent a house, find a school. Perhaps she might come and live in Stroud? We look at possible schools but I already know she'll go to Hay-on-Wye. She fell in love with it during her road trip over the summer.

She's been on a yoga retreat in Wales, is lithe and weightless, eats nothing. She's acquired a red, second-hand ballerina-type dress and floats through Stroud, immediately making friends in a way that I will entirely fail to do. Men fancy her and I am jealous. She's creating a new life, emerging from her chrysalis, spreading damp and brightly coloured wings.

Of course, the reality is quite different. She's a single mother with no money and nowhere to live. And she's now locked in a nasty battle about money with her ex-husband. But still she manages to make her life look free, lightweight. We talk about the fact that we are both living too fast, trying to do too many things.

If I don't stop, I say, something awful will happen.

Yes. Like getting cancer or something.

But neither of us can stop.

I just didn't know, Joslin says, how much courage would be required for a fairly normal life.

The world financial system is in meltdown. Every day the newspaper headlines suggest that one or more of the major UK banks will collapse. But still autumn glimmers golden, day after long day. In the mornings the sun hangs low and red over the road that leads across Rodborough Common. Threads of mist stretch across the grass. Occasional golfers appear like ghosts beside the road, cows the size of vans congregate at Tom Long's Post, causing traffic chaos. I'm up early every morning, driving that road, taking Thomas to school.

Sometimes, on my way back, I stop the car in one of the National Trust car parks, open the door and get out, watch my breath rise in white clouds around me, sit on the warm bonnet of the car, so I can see the day unfolding. The mist clears revealing hills, farms and cottages, organised on distant ledges. I'm on top of the world here, quite alone. To one side the long stretches of the Cotswold Hills, reaching all the way to Oxford, and on the other the Severn Vale, low-lying and damp, edging that least friendly of rivers.

It's on a morning like this, when I'm propped against the car bonnet, wrapped in my coat, that the truth appears. Or at least a new life-saving cliché emerges. In a sudden blooming of light, I see it all with frightening clarity. I know completely and absolutely what's happened to us. The facts are startlingly apparent, lit in neon in my mind. Advertised for all to see, beyond argument.

We've lost four babies in the space of four years. We've been let down by the medical profession and we won't ever have another living child. This is the situation. *This didn't happen to someone else, it happened to me.* When my Norwegian friend made that statement I didn't understand. Now it seems both so obvious as to be not worth making, and so profound that it explains everything.

And there's no meaning to be found in this, no path towards greater wisdom. Why does the same thing keep happening again and again? If the Almighty exists, and if He has been trying to teach me a lesson, then clearly He thinks I'm stone deaf. No, all of that is just a mental construct that may once have been useful but is now a burden. What's happened is simply what's happened, nothing more. Now that I see this, the choices are also startlingly clear. I could lie down and die. Except that I already know that you can lie down for a long time and you won't die. In order to die, you have to do something drastic and I don't have the energy for that. And so I'm destined to stay here, alive.

And perhaps life isn't so bad after all. I have my son and my husband and we're starting a new life. All I need to do is to find some small thing to enjoy in the day. And actually there's plenty of pleasure on offer – particularly in this early morning moment. The dog walkers setting out across the Common, a bright red kite which, even at this early hour, swoops and flaps through the high white air.

And now the mist rises higher and the sun comes through more clearly and the whole of the Severn Vale is revealed below. I feel a great weight lifting from me. It's such a relief – such an incredible relief – to understand that this is all quite random. No meaning, no lessons, no point to anything. Just find one small thing to enjoy in the day.

Stephen decides that we should give away our money – or at least any money that we don't need for the house renovations. Over the years Stephen has acquired money by being an exceptional lawyer, but he never planned to make more than a reasonable salary. Now as the pay cheques roll in he shrugs his shoulders and says – I just don't need any more Marks and Spencer lambswool V-neck jumpers.

Maybe there's a course on How to Be Rich? I say. Do you think if you signed up, you would get the hang of it?

In Brussels, it was easy to ignore the money. No one there knows what anyone earns, which is one of the reasons why we liked living there. But in England it isn't so simple. And the money does seem important now in a way that it never has before. It's something we still have on our side.

Just give it away, Stephen says, and I agree.

And it sounds easy – but we are soon lost in the philanthropy supermarket. Stephen is frustrated. He wants to get rid of the money right now. People need it – what's the point in delaying? I agree but still we dither.

Then Stephen meets new friends who can help and finds charities he wants to support, encounters people who inspire him. I don't consider what we're doing to be good, only logical. Good people are those on low incomes, who work long hours and still give to charity or do voluntary work. For us, giving is easy. It isn't morally right, only logical.

What we need is an end to our story and this could be just what we are looking for. *Yes, they lived through such a difficult time but then they raised all this money for charity.* It all sounds so easy and tempting but somehow, although I'm glad to give the money away, it doesn't provide the sense of resolution that I need.

Stephen objects to the idea that we've given away our money because Laura died. He says we'd have done the same anyway – sometime. That may be true but I still feel sure that we can relate to other people's suffering more fully now. I don't believe any more in finding the gifts of grief – but, if I did, this might be one of them.

Barack Obama is elected President of the United States. The days keep coming at me. Some can be managed, some cannot. Everyone in this new life asks the same question – just the one child then? And I curve my lips upwards, make my eyes bright and say – Yes, just the one. I do this because Stephen and I've agreed that, since we're starting a new life, we're not going to tell many people. Or certainly not initially.

Stephen says that people find it off-putting to be told this kind of information when they first meet someone. We don't want to be pitiful any more, we don't want to look like victims. We don't want people to smell death on us and decide that they don't need our tragedy in their lives.

To begin with I do quite well at pretending. Just the one child then? Yes, just the one. It's such a harmless question. Before Laura died I probably often asked that question myself. But soon I'm at the stage when I stop going out of the house, avoid talking to anyone, because I don't want to be asked that question. What I fear beyond anything else is kindness.

The school is the worst. Little girls in green-and-blue-checked dresses play with skipping ropes. Their hair is held back by green bands and their plaits bounce as they jump. One day a little girl runs across my path and she's wearing Laura's coat – that navy blue coat, fitted at the waist, with a rounded velvet collar and velvet-covered buttons. Her silver-blonde hair is cut bluntly and falls to just above her shoulders. Her legs are thin as wire and her woollen tights wrinkle at the ankle. I hurry back to the car, with my head down. On the way home I stop on the Common, lean my head on the steering wheel for a while.

I need to talk, to say something to someone. I don't need to tell them the whole story, to cry and be comforted. I just want to state the fact, that's all. I can't just keep going in and out of the school with my teeth gritted and my head down. Just the one child then? Oh yes, you've got the little girl in reception, haven't you? No, no. I don't have a little girl. Yes, the tiny blonde girl. No. No.

A day arrives when I can't do it any more and so I promise myself that I'll say something to someone. Just state the fact, that's all. The first person who says – Just the one child? I'll tell that person. Just say the words. It can't be so bad. The sky will not fall down – or it shouldn't.

The corridor to Thomas's classroom is crowded. Mums and dads push through, picking up fleeces and school bags. The walls are decorated with wax crayon pictures of dinosaurs and a high-up shelf is crowded with clay models and sausage dogs made out of the inside of loo rolls. I find myself pressed up against a woman with blonde hair and a kindly smile.

You new here?

Yes.

Oh right. And who've you got then?

Thomas. In Miss Betts' class.

Oh right. Just the one then?

Yes. No. I had another. I had a little girl, but she was born dead.

Silence drops like a blanket over us. Even in the crowded school corridor.

Oh my God. I'm sorry. Oh. So did I – a little boy. Anthony. I've Harry and David – alive – but there was Anthony. Died in the womb, thirty-two weeks.

I stand there staring at her. How does this happen? I picked this woman at random and yet she's the woman who also had a stillborn baby. Are there many more women than I realise? Or, at some strange level, when you see someone do you know? We stand in the corridor staring at each other and I feel tears forming.

Come back, she says. Come back and have some tea.

And so Thomas and I go back to Anna's house, opposite the church in Amberley and she tells me about Anthony. She has a photograph of Anthony but she doesn't show him to many people. By the time they got him out he didn't look how he should have done.

She shows me the photograph. Thomas and her boys play out in the garden.

You do get it all, don't you? she says. A woman I knew at that time said to me – I know exactly what you're going through because my greyhound died.

She pours more tea, discovers that I'm a writer.

You should write it down, she says.

I don't think so.

Yes, you know. Misery memoir. All the rage, aren't they?

Yes. But nobody is interested in a talking wound. Even a misery memoir has a happy ending. That's the whole point of them. Adversity overcome. There isn't any place in our world for stories that don't have happy endings – despite the fact that those stories are all around us.

Yeah, she says. You're right.

All onward and upward, I say. Positive thinking. Which, paradoxically, is probably why there is so much depression around the place.

Anna goes to call the boys in for tea, returns.

I think for me the worst thing is that I used to be someone that people were jealous of, Anna says. People wanted my life. Now they look at me and just thank their lucky stars it wasn't them.

The boys shout out in the garden.

But I was lucky, she says. I had three close friends at that time and I just sat at their kitchen tables day after day after day and talked on and on and on about what happened. Mind you, all three of them have emigrated now.

XV

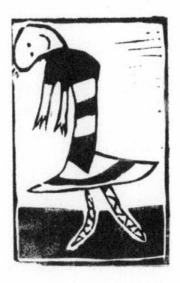

If we could read the secret history of our enemies,
we should find in each man's life sorrow and
suffering enough to disarm all hostility.

Henry Wadsworth Longfellow

So here we are with our new lives and I'm making it work. Autumn has faded. It's colder here than in Brussels but there's more light. I've made up my mind. If I can't have a second child then that means that my life is intended for some other purpose. I just need to wait and that purpose will become clear. Perhaps I'll become a famous writer, or a war reporter, or maybe I'll just travel the world writing about everything I see – and Thomas will come with me. I'm looking forward to cutting myself loose from the world of babies and mother-hood – a world where I have so abjectly failed, a world which never interested me anyway.

And then I get pregnant again. I find out at five o'clock on a November afternoon. Mercifully Thomas has gone to play with a friend. I pull a chair up close to the Aga and ring Joslin in Hay-on-Wye. You're an urban myth, she says. You know those stories – the woman who did IVF ten times, was in the process of adopting.

I know. I've given all my baby stuff away. The Big Man in the sky does like a joke, doesn't He? And I'm not sure His jokes are always in very good taste.

But it is good news?

Oh yes. Even if I have another miscarriage, I'm glad. I know that the odds are badly stacked against us but at least some-thing has happened, at least I've got another chance.

All the family are due to come to Mount Vernon for Christ-mas. A family conference hastily decides that Christmas will go ahead as planned but that I'm to do nothing. I'd been dreading all the Christmas preparations and so I'm pleased to find myself relieved of all responsibility. Stephen is thrilled that we have another chance.

I book to go to the doctor's. I've never been to the surgery in Stroud before and so I have to tell the whole ugly story. The doctor tells me to speak to the receptionist and she will make the necessary appointments at the local hospital. I walk up to the desk and the receptionist says – Congratulations. When is the baby due?

Listen, I lost the last four. It's not helpful for me to have this conversation.

But the receptionist needs to know. All of her calculations and plans depend on that date. She hands me a pile of brochures and booklets. One contains a full plan of all the stages of the pregnancy, advice on indigestion and piles, endless adverts for baby slings, cots, maternity bras, little bells you can hang around your neck so the baby hears them in the womb.

I walk out of the surgery even though the receptionist is only halfway through the forms. When I get home I drop all the leaflets straight in the recycling. I can't afford to make even the smallest emotional investment in this. I can cope with despair but not with hope.

This time I'm determined we're going to get some decent medical help, someone who will give us proper information, who will care about what happens to us. Every other woman I know who has had a stillbirth has been referred to a specialist unit for problem pregnancies, but that never happens to me. To be fair, this is because we've moved hospitals, moved country. But now I'm not waiting around for someone to offer help. I do some research and find a consultant at the John Radcliffe Hospital in Oxford and book an appointment to see him in January.

The family come for Christmas. Everyone congratulates me. I don't remember anything much about Christmas. My mum and my West London aunt make it all happen despite the ruined state of the house. I realise that I don't feel pregnant any more and find that I'm bleeding slightly, but I don't say anything because I don't want to ruin Christmas.

Everyone is leaving on Boxing Day and I decide I'll ring the hospital then. So after lunch I go upstairs to the empty and undecorated sitting room and phone the out-of-hours GP service. They tell me that because of the holiday period, I will have to wait three days until I can have an appointment. At that appointment they will assess whether I need to go to Gloucester Hospital for a scan. I explain my situation but they can offer nothing more.

So what if I just go now to Gloucester Hospital and ask for a scan?

No, you can't do that. They won't see you unless we refer you.

I am white with rage. I understand that it's Boxing Day. I understand that, from their point of view, I'm just suffering a miscarriage, and that happens every day. But surely my medical history is going to make it possible for them to help me? Apparently not.

I wave goodbye to the family but my sister stays on. We talk about what I should do. She says that if Gloucester Hospital won't see me then we should go to Cheltenham instead. I agree but I can't ask Stephen, I can't see him suffer any more. And I don't want Thomas to know what is happening, I want him to have his Happy Christmas. My sister says immediately that she will drive me there.

Casualty at Cheltenham Hospital is empty. My sister and I sit waiting amidst the buzzing coffee machines, the tired Christmas decorations and the drooping racks of leaflets.

Disasters should at least involve variety, novelty, surprise. Eventually I'm called to the desk and I say that I want to have a scan. The lady I speak to explains that I will have to wait forty-eight hours. I lose my cool.

I'm not leaving this hospital until I have a scan.

She says she will go and find someone to talk to me.

My sister and I wait another hour. Eventually a nurse beckons me into a private office.

Let me get you some paracetamol, she says.

No thank you. I'm not in pain.

Oh right. She takes out a form and writes down details.

Oh dear, she says. Oh dear. Are you sure you don't want some paracetamol?

No thank you. She stares at me in an intense, doe-eyed way. I don't understand what this is about. Finally I conclude that the look is meant to convey deep sympathy but I don't want sympathy, I just want a scan. I just want to know whether the baby is dead or alive.

OK, I say. So what about tomorrow?

Apparently that won't be possible.

Are there any scans taking place tomorrow? I ask.

Oh yes, there are. But you see those are all scheduled scans. They've all been booked in.

And they can't fit in one extra?

No. The schedule is very tight.

I've gone past anger now and into exhaustion, but still I keep going. I need to have a scan. I'm not prepared to wait. What is the solution? Are you sure you don't need some paracetamol? Best to take it with a glass of water.

Finally the nurse promises that if I go home someone from the maternity ward will ring me later. My sister drives me home. I enter the house, open the sitting room door. Thomas and Stephen are on the floor, assembling Thomas's new Lego ship. Stephen and I don't speak. He already knows that the hospital will not help us. I go upstairs without turning the light on, feel the darkness of the house around me, pull off my clothes, get into bed.

I lie awake all night, alive with anger. No call comes from the hospital. The next morning I wake early and Stephen and I decide that we'll go back to the hospital. We have no choice but to take Thomas but Stephen's mum offers to pick him up from there and look after him. At the hospital, we wait in Casualty. When I'm called over to the desk, it's revealed that no message reached the maternity ward last night. I am told once again that no scan can be arranged for another forty-eight hours. I start to shout and keep shouting.

A nurse appears and offers paracetamol. I am causing embarrassment and so am shuffled into a side room. Assurances are offered that someone will be coming to see me soon. A frightened young trainee arrives and takes my blood pressure. I know that she's just been sent to waste time and I shout at her and then regret it. Eventually a real doctor arrives and agrees that I can have a scan. Suddenly everyone seems concerned.

So this is an IVF baby?

It's clear that if I answer yes then I will be taken seriously.

No. No. It's the baby after the IVF failed.

That seems of less interest. I am taken to a corridor where Stephen and I wait for the scan. The door to the scanning room opens and I see darkness, lights from a machine, black and white images flickering on a screen. My mind plunges into fear and then the door shuts again and I steady myself. Finally we are called. I say to the lady operating the equipment that I'm pretty sure that the baby is dead. Neither

Stephen nor I look at the screen or ask any questions. Our fears are confirmed.

Afterwards I ask the doctor if I can have a D and C. I don't want to see blood or anything that might ever have been the beginnings of a baby. The doctor is sympathetic but full of blather about the reasons why this isn't a good idea. She doesn't say anything about money but I know that's what this is about.

Let's discuss all this when things get back to normal. Just wait three months and then we can discuss the next pregnancy.

More paracetamol is offered. Stephen and I leave the hospital.

I'm lying in bed and Thomas is next to me. It's ten o'clock at night. I'm in pain and I can't sleep but there is no blood. I don't understand why that is but I can't face ringing the hospital. It's bitterly cold but we haven't got any heating on. The house is so badly insulated that the heating costs a fortune and doesn't make any difference. Thomas can't sleep and so we're listening to the Narnia books on an audio CD. Stephen is downstairs, drinking red wine, messing around on the computer. Eventually, Thomas drifts into sleep and Stephen comes upstairs and sits on the bed.

Did you know it's New Year?

Is it? Oh. Yes, I did hear fireworks but I never thought.

I didn't know either, he says. But I just put the radio on.

I'm shocked to realise how totally cut off from the rest of the world we've become, up here in our half-ruined house. How is it possible not to know that it's New Year? Somewhere not far away there are people having parties and letting off fireworks.

Perhaps we should put the radio on and listen to the New Year being rung in? I suggest.

Should we?

No, perhaps not. I don't think I can be bothered.

Stephen gets into bed next to Thomas and me. They sleep and I lie awake, listening.

Joslin arrives from Hay-on-Wye with Matthew. Her relationship with Matthew has amicably disintegrated and she's now going out with Wayland, Matthew's close friend, so he stays as well. They come like a circus – all bright colours and fun. Thomas, Ellie and James run through the ruins of the house, playing hide and seek. Then they whizz down the drive in Thomas's Christmas present go-cart. Joslin, Matthew and Wayland seem high on new friendship, hope for the future.

I can't see or hear or speak. I may always have been the Spectre at the Feast – the person who watched rather than participated. But now I don't even watch. I am separated from my friends by frosted glass, but still I try to play the game, although my movements are stilted, my voice hoarse. I tell them that I've been trying to work out how we could get Laura's rose bush from the garden of the house in Brussels and bring it home. They acknowledge that this is important and Stephen agrees, but I know it won't happen. We all go out for the evening into Stroud. In a café poems are read, guitars played. People sing and dance. I escape and wander through the icy, deserted town. Eventually I prop myself on a low wall, lean my head against another wall, wait until everyone is ready to go home.

My friends care, of course, I know they do. But I'm far beyond reach.

But, as ever, things are not as they seem. Only a few days

after Joslin leaves, she notices that Ellie isn't walking well. She knows immediately that the situation is serious and she is right. Ellie has a rare condition called Guillain-Barré Syndrome and is immediately taken into hospital. If the progress of the disease can't be halted, she will die. For two or three days, life stops, everyone waits, hopes. Finally the treatment works but still her recovery period will be long and she'll have difficulty walking for many months. Joslin sends a picture which Ellie has drawn of herself – a collapsing woman, crooked and floppy, limp. It seems like an image that carries a larger message. Why are the women all falling? Always falling?

A few days later the snow is thick on the ground and our lane is coated with ice so I can't move the car. Stephen is away in Brussels. A red sun hangs low in the sky. I'm meant to be going to the hospital but can't get there. I'm glad about that. The hours stretch ahead, endlessly. The snow brings with it a fragile silence. The white cold presses in on the house, the hills. I don't see or speak to anyone. I don't answer the phone. It's easier like that.

Although the pregnancy has failed, we still have an appointment to go and see the consultant at the John Radcliffe. I don't want to go but, when Stephen comes back from Brussels, he insists and so we set off for Oxford. The snow has cleared but it rains heavily all the way there. It's been raining for three years now.

The appointment with the consultant is all about statistics. If you've lost five babies then the chance that you'll lose another is 50 per cent. If you get pregnant at forty-two then you have a 50 per cent chance of losing the baby. If you have had a detached placenta then there's a 10 per cent chance it will happen again, but the risk is much higher if you are older.

As I'm not much good at maths, I am uncertain whether one of these figures is subsumed into the others, or whether I am meant to add them all together. If the latter is true then I seem to have at least a 110 per cent chance of losing another baby. In another mood I might see the comic side of this. The consultant is doing his best. But soon I stop listening. Even I can figure out that, no matter how you add the figures up, the answer always equals Totally and Utterly Hopeless.

The consultant says that he's prepared to try and do IVF again for us, but there is a waiting list. He asks us if we've thought about the possibility of donor eggs. I have recently read a couple of articles in the papers about this but I don't really know what it means. He explains that I could be implanted with an egg from another woman, a donor, and that would increase the chances of success. But we would have almost no chance of getting a donor egg in the UK.

Couples who want to pursue this option usually have to go to Spain or America. He gives us the details of a clinic in Spain. I'm angry with Stephen for even discussing this because he knows I don't want to do it. No more medical treatment, no more hospitals.

How about surrogacy? Stephen says.

Oh no, no, no, no, the consultant says. That's a disaster. Certainly not.

I just want to get out of his office. So far I have managed not to cry or say bitter things but soon I will lose control. As we leave the consultant's office he says – You know there's a café, if you want a cup of tea. At the end of the corridor, a cup of tea.

Poor man, we want a baby and all he can offer is a cup of tea.

And that's how I remember him, the senior consultant at the John Radcliffe, a man in a corridor, gesturing as though explaining something to the deaf or partially sighted. You can have a cup of tea. This way – the café. Arms waving, smiles, enthusiasm. The glaring light in the corridor, all that hushed plate glass. Yes, yes. A cup of tea.

Then I get a letter from Joslin. She has written to me because she doesn't feel able to call. She's pregnant again and she just isn't sure she wants to be pregnant. Because of me, because she's really not in a situation where she can bring up a new baby. Because Ellie is sick and in a wheelchair. Because her relationship is so new. Because so much of her time and energy are being taken up by nasty negotiations with her ex-husband. She knows I will be angry, she herself is confused and worried. She wants so much for us always to be friends but she understands if I don't want to talk to her.

It takes me a week to call. We manage to laugh. These strange coincidences between her life and mine. She is sure now that the pregnancy is fine, all for the best. I agree because what else can I do? She says that really she does want another child. I'm the wrong person to be talking to her and we both know it. I can't be objective, I can't rise above my own situation. I don't understand why, when her life is already complicated, she has made it yet more complicated. But of course, we are still friends, always will be.

I decide that now that I'm back in England I'm going to go to a stillbirth support group. That's something I could never do in Brussels. I get in touch with the lady who runs the group in Bristol and she is called Janey. She says I'm very welcome to come along.

Bristol is forty minutes away and I dread the journey because I'm not good at driving in places which I don't know at night – but still I'm determined to go. Typically I make the situation worse by failing to print off a map before I leave. And so I spend hours driving around the suburbs, lost and increasingly desperate.

All the while Janey is sending me texts and trying to help me get there. Eventually I arrive at a community centre in a tangle of some backstreets. And there is Janey – on her own. She usually has more people turning up, she tells me. But I'm the first person to come tonight. She always sits there all evening anyway because you can never tell who might come, or when.

She's a tall, thin woman, with lovely long black hair. She's dignified, resolute and calm, sitting here on her own, in this nowhere place. She's here to help women who've lost babies, despite the fact that she has an awful story to tell herself. She's waving a flag for the bereaved, which is something that few people do.

Probably it's best that there's just the two of us, she tells me. That means we can talk properly. Also … well, of course, there's quite a group of bereaved mums who are expecting again. They would be very happy to welcome you but I don't know how you would feel about that.

I consider her question. I don't think that the pregnant women would bother me but I suspect that I would bother them. Even in this group I can't be totally at home.

I set up the group, Janey tells me. Because I felt I owed it to our lost son, Oliver.

She stares out of the window briefly.

I don't want to boast, she says. It's no big deal. But overall I feel I've done him proud.

No words are needed.

You have done, Janey. You have.

After the meeting, I set out to drive home. It's a straight run up the motorway from Bristol to Stroud but I get lost, totally lost. I can't find the motorway. I keep taking one turn after another – right, left, right – leaving the city behind, plunging into country lanes, sure that soon I must come to a place I recognise, but I seem to be going around in circles. At one moment, I even glimpse the lights looping along the motorway but I can't get there. I should stop but I can't. I can only keep driving, on and on, one turn after another, digging my way deeper and deeper into the blackness of nowhere.

Eventually I stop. The night is dark all around me. There is no moon, no light from a star or a distant street lamp. The road is a nondescript country road, deserted, with not a car or house in sight. I sit staring out of the window ahead of me, shivering. Then I get out of the car and open the boot to find the map – but there is no map.

I look up at the starless night. And suddenly I understand that I am lost – not just lost somewhere in the countryside outside Bristol – but completely lost. Connected to nothing and no one, cut loose somewhere in the infinite night. I have taken a road that no one else has taken. I am in a world without maps. Even in the grim context of The Dead Baby Club I am not truly welcome. All that is left to me now is a sense of myself as being – miraculously – still alive.

XVI

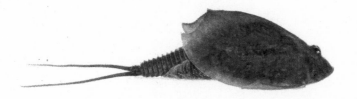

'Life ... is a tale told by an idiot, full of
sound and fury, signifying nothing.'

William Shakespeare, *MacBeth*

So – adoption. I'd always wanted to adopt and now that we're back in the UK then surely that might be possible? This is what we should have done as soon as Laura died. But Stephen isn't convinced by the adoption idea. This doesn't surprise me because I've already spoken to a number of couples who have considered adoption, and it seems that often whereas a woman just wants a baby, a man wants to carry on his genetic line. I'm grateful to Stephen for considering the question despite his reservations.

Of course, the decision is not entirely ours. Thomas's happiness has to be our priority. Stephen and I agree with ease that colour or race isn't an issue. Chinese, Russian, Ethiopian, Thai – all of that is possible. I fantasise about a tiny Asian girl, black hair in pigtails secured by plastic bobbles. But age? That's more complicated. Thomas has lost his sister. Is it fair to bring a four-year-old child into his life, particularly as that child might have emotional difficulties?

We think not. Are we using Thomas's needs as a way of hiding our own desires and prejudices? Yes, probably. But Stephen and I are no longer the people we were four years ago. We have had our own tragedies and so feel less able to take on other people's difficulties. Doubtless that is selfish of us.

In reality, however, decisions about what kind of child we might adopt are the least of our worries. First we have to be approved for adoption and we know that this is a major hurdle. In my mind, a fantasy scene plays again and again. Late on a rainy winter's night a knock sounds at the front door. A woman in a black coat holds a bundle wrapped in her arms. Please, she says. Please. This baby – it needs a home. Can you take it? Will you look after it?

And I stretch out my arms and take the baby. No questions asked. Yes, of course, I'll look after this baby, or any baby. Yes, of course. You can trust me absolutely. The baby will be happy with us. If only it could be this simple.

I call Gloucestershire County Council who explain that their adoption services are contracted out to an agency called Child First. I call Child First but no one rings back. Eventually I find information on the internet about an evening seminar and I sign up. This seminar takes place in a church hall somewhere in West Oxford. About forty people are in the audience. Sitting among these other couples, I'm preoccupied once again by the hierarchies of grief. Presumably, the vast majority here are people who, for whatever reason, will never have a child of their own.

I'll play – five Dead Babies in four years.

I'll raise you – no possibility of ever having a child of our own.

They lay down their final ace, as they must. We are lucky, I know that. But we never find out anything about any of these other couples because it soon becomes apparent that no one in this room is allowed a story, a past.

A couple who have already adopted have been brought along to tell the story of how they became parents to four-year-old twins from an abusive background. Their story is heart-warming and inspiring but they never give any details of why they adopted. Is this not an essential part of their story? Also, they never say whether they have ever felt any grief about not having children who are genetically theirs. And somehow everyone in the room knows not to ask.

After they have spoken, a social worker stands beside a whiteboard and explains the process, drawing endless incomprehensible diagrams of boxes and twisting lines. I look around at the other couples. Their eyes are blank, puzzled. Some start to yawn while others scratch their heads. The social worker has become a tic-tac man at a racecourse, frantically waving her arms, speaking a language which no one understands. We all start to stare at our shoes.

A man in the audience is trying to raise his hand but his wife keeps pulling his arm back down. He refuses to be silenced – So any sixteen-year-old girl can go into an alleyway on Saturday night, he says. And have a knee-trembler with a bloke whose name she doesn't know and no one is ever going to ask about her suitability for motherhood. But I'm going to have to go through all this just to be a father?

The room is silent. The man's wife is tearful. A social worker crouching in the corner makes a note in her black book. We all know that this couple have fallen at the first hurdle. And yet this man has only said what everyone in the room is thinking.

After the seminar I ring Child First again and a time is fixed for a social worker to talk to me. She rings up and informs me that no babies are available for adoption in England. The only children available for adoption are at least three years old and most of them have disabilities or severe emotional difficulties.

I ask about overseas adoption. The social worker doesn't seem keen to discuss this. If I want to know about overseas adoption then I will need to speak to others who have been through that experience. She warns me that the process is long, difficult and expensive. Of course, she tells me, living in rural Gloucestershire, you wouldn't be able to adopt a black or mixed-race child.

Oh right.

I think of two white couples we know in Brussels who have adopted children who are black or Asian. The first time I met those families I noted that the children must be adopted but then never thought about it again. No one in Brussels does think of it because mixed-race adoption is relatively common. In England it's seen as a problem and, therefore, it doesn't exist. And so it is a problem. Chicken and egg. But it isn't going to help if I argue with the social worker.

China used to be a good bet, she says, if you want a girl. But now that country is closing down. Many people have been trying to adopt from there for years without success.

Oh right. And Russia?

I've already done my research and know that Russia is probably our best bet.

Well, yes, she says. Yes. I suppose that might be your only option really. But, of course, most of the babies have foetal alcohol syndrome. And the process takes at least four years. Also, you said that you are forty-three and your husband is nearly fifty. Well, once he is fifty then he will be too old to adopt.

Oh right. I see.

She clearly isn't going to give me any more information. End of call.

I often think now about Jacobean drama and, in particular, Thomas Middleton's play *The Revenger's Tragedy*. It's a play that is seldom performed because, in the last act, nearly every character dies, is murdered or commits suicide. And, as the bodies pile up, the audience usually starts to titter in embarrassment, then to laugh uproariously.

I feel that I'm now living in a performance of that play. I can't talk to people about what has happened because they can't take it in. My story demands too much of the listener, no response that he or she might make is appropriate. If you have too much death then it becomes silly. A thing of cardboard swords, blood pellets and theatrical groans of agony. And that makes people laugh. I also find myself inwardly laughing because it's the only reaction left to me.

We discover that we have thirty thousand bees living on the roof of the house. A man who knows about bees comes with equipment to begin the process of moving them. He lifts a honeycomb which is taller than Thomas from one of the chimneys on the tower. Thomas and I watch from the lawn, fascinated and a little unnerved.

Next morning I open the door of the shower room to find it black with bees. Confused by the intervention of the bee man, they have moved down the chimney and come into the shower room through an old ventilation shaft. Stephen is away and I am uncertain who to call. The police? The fire brigade?

Finally I put on a long mackintosh, and gloves, cover my face with a scarf. If I can get across the bathroom to the window and open it then maybe the bees will leave. My plan works and most of the bees fly out of the window and back up to the tower. Hastily I block the ventilation shaft with tape.

Now that we are in the country there is an awful lot of reproduction. A friend on the school run is struggling with gerbils who won't stop reproducing. She takes them to the vet to try to get some of them destroyed but it costs £30 per gerbil. Finally she has to release a load of them onto the Common because she just doesn't know what to do with them.

Then Thomas gets head lice – again and again. And we

decide to go in for Triops, which are tiny creatures like miniature dinosaurs that breed in water. It's meant to be easy to
breed them but we only ever get one, whom we name Finny.
Too many gerbils and head lice, too few Triops. Reproduction
isn't tidily organised. I worry about Finny. Thomas is thrilled
with him but he still wants the hamster he was promised when
we were leaving Brussels.

Darling, I'm sorry. I just can't deal with things dying.

It's all right, Mummy. It'll be fine. We'll just dig a grave and
make a cross and sing a hymn and it will all be fine.

But still I fail to get a hamster.

I contact an organisation which specialises in advising on
overseas adoption and we sign up for another seminar. It
takes place in Barnet in North London in rooms over a shop.
Again about twenty couples attend. We are made to play a
bizarre board game. Adoption Monopoly? Or is it Snakes and
Ladders but without any Ladders? Each couple has a marker
to move around the board. Cards are drawn from a pack.
They say – *Your paperwork has been lost, go back three
months.* Or – *The country you have chosen is now closed for
adoption, go back to square one.*

It comes to our turn. So Stephen and Alice, where are you
up to now?

Well, I've just retired, Stephen says, pretending to read the
card.

No one dares laugh or it'll be back to the beginning for
them.

After that they show us a film about overseas adoption.
Images appear of an orphanage in India – row upon row of
tiny, shrunken babies lie in cots which look more like cages,
and their thin little voices wail. Panic starts in my toes and

rises swiftly through my body, bringing with it breathlessness and nausea. I'm up and out of the room, standing out in a grey carpeted corridor, my head pressed against a frosted glass window. Why do those orphanages exist when a whole room full of couples here would be happy to give those babies a home? I try to remind myself that it isn't as simple as that.

We break for a coffee and chat to the lady running the seminar. We ask her if it is possible for us to begin to try to adopt in the UK and, if that proves impossible, move on to the overseas option. No, that isn't possible. The two processes are entirely different and if you want to move from one to the other then you have to start again. And, in fact, if you are given permission to adopt from overseas then that permission relates to one country only. So if you try to adopt from China and that fails and you decide to try Russia instead, then once again you go back to the beginning of the process.

We nod and smile, move on and speak to some of the other couples, hoping to find just a word or two of encouragement. One couple can't currently be considered for adoption because, although they are homeowners and employed, they have £5,000 of credit card debt. Another couple used to live in Bedfordshire, and they got two years into the adoption process, but then they moved to Berkshire so they had to begin again.

After coffee the discussion focuses on the difficulties experienced by adopted children. Two men interrupt – one is black, the other of Asian origin. Both of them were themselves adopted. The lady running the seminar is clearly uncomfortable with real-life multicultural adoption stories. But she presses them to express the anger they must surely feel towards their adoptive parents.

Anger? I was in an orphanage in Thailand and my mum and dad adopted me, brought me back here, gave me everything. From an early age I wanted to be a musician and they made that possible. How could I possibly be angry?

Then the black guy says – I was adopted from Ghana and for me it was certainly traumatic. Because every year my adoptive family in Hampstead wanted to celebrate Ghanaian National Day. So all my flabby, white relatives dressed up in African costumes and played drums. Man, I've been on the psychiatrist's couch for years.

Doubtless the names of these two have gone into the black book as well.

I haven't spoken to Joslin for a couple of months. The news isn't good. She has terrible pains in her back but no one seems to be able to tell her why. The doctors say it's just because this is the third pregnancy and she has two other children to look after. And on top of that, there's the stress of Ellie's illness. A week later I get a text from Joslin saying that she has had to go into hospital because the pain is just too bad. The hospital can't find anything wrong and send her home again but the pain isn't much better. Joslin texts to say that at least Ellie is walking again now. I don't really know how to respond.

After further awkward conversations with Child First, I manage to book an appointment for us to talk to a social worker in person. This appointment will last for two hours and after that it may be possible for us to begin the process. As Stephen and I set out for the meeting I get a text from Wayland telling me that Joslin is in hospital again with back pains and I promise myself I'll call her later. Our meeting takes place in a room with comfy chairs, sash windows looking onto the street. A box of tissues has thoughtfully been provided but there is no saucepan for bashing on the floor.

The social worker is middle-aged with blonde hair, weepy eyes, baggy clothes, a chunky necklace. She views us with manufactured sympathy and concern, reassures us that we can be quite honest and open. To me this statement seems in itself dishonest. She holds all the power and she is judging us. That's the nature of this process so wouldn't it be better to admit that?

Initially the discussion seems to go quite well. I've been to see plenty of shrinks and so I know what to say. I even begin to feel a little guilty about how successfully I am manipulating this discussion. But soon I begin to notice that the social worker finds problems everywhere. I talk about Thomas because he's surely the best card we have to play.

The good thing is that he is older, I say. So fewer problems with sibling rivalry.

Oh no, the social worker says. You'll have serious problems. Of course.

I'm thinking – surely sibling rivalry isn't really a problem, just a fact of family life? But I keep my mouth shut, as I must. And so it goes on. No and no and no. We are guilty until proven innocent. This encounter is turning into a scene from *The Trial* by Kafka. We have to convince this woman that we want a child, but it's clear that we must not appear to want one too much.

Of course, we have to tell the story of Laura, of the miscarriages, the IVF. The social worker thinks we have too much baggage, asks various intrusive questions about our grief. I'm being pushed to say that I never think of Laura now. But I'm not going to say that. Instead I say that Laura travels with us, that she's part of our lives and always will be but that we try to make her a source of happiness and love rather than sadness. This clearly isn't enough.

And living abroad, the social worker says. You don't have a settled community in the UK.

I want to say – listen, please, can't you see that this isn't Plan A? Neither is it Plan B, C, D, E or F. But we're trying to look to the future, to find some hope, to forge a way forward in difficult circumstances. Could you at least try to meet us halfway? But the social worker doesn't care about us because her job is just to take care of the interests of children who need to be adopted. That's all very well but is she going to help those children by browbeating us?

Actually, I think we do have a pretty strong community in the UK, Stephen says. Alice's mother and sister live nearby. My parents live less than half an hour away, as do my two brothers, their wives and my nieces.

The social worker eyes him as if he's trying to cause trouble.

Then it comes out that Stephen and I were both at boarding school. The social worker makes no attempt to hide the fact that she considers us to be gravely psychologically damaged. She asks us why we went to boarding school. Stephen explains that his father was in the Air Force and moved every two years and so he went away to school for reasons of stability. I could invent some similar reason to explain my family's choices but I'm getting bored by this and I'm angry that someone in a position of power should flaunt their prejudices so openly.

Actually, I just went to boarding school for social reasons. That's just what my family do.

The social worker shrugs, purses her lips as though she's tasted something nasty.

We're asked if either of us smoke. Stephen is also bored and angry now.

Yeah, actually, he says. I do.

No, I say. No. It's not really like that. About once every

three months Stephen goes out late and has a few glasses of wine and then he has one cigarette. He never smokes at home, never has.

The social worker ignores me and turns to Stephen – So you smoke?

Once every three months, yes.

She fixes Stephen with a glare that could strip paint.

Well, I suggest you stop.

But finally it isn't the one cigarette that finishes us, or Thomas, or our past history. Instead it's the fact that we're about to have building work done in our house.

But wait a minute, Stephen says. You've just told us that this process will take years and the building work is only scheduled to take three months.

This makes no difference, apparently. We can't start the process of being approved for adoption until our building work is finished. And even after that we may not be able to start because it's possible that no social worker will be available to work with us. Stephen and I nod pleasantly although we're both stunned. The meeting comes to an amicable end and we agree that we'll get back in touch when the building work is finished. I shake the social worker's clammy hand, force myself to smile.

But as we drive home, Stephen is fuming and I am in tears. I know the social worker is playing games, trying to find out if we are serious. But could she not have offered some support or encouragement? I know that adoption isn't easy – and that it shouldn't be. But would they really rather leave one hundred children in care than relax their impossible demands for perfection? I convince myself that this is a minor setback. We'll just wait until the building work is finished and then we'll press ahead. But in reality I know that we're in the process of losing yet another child, this time a tiny Asian girl with black pigtails held up by plastic bobbles. At home I comfort myself by reading R. S. Thomas. Time is a main road, eternity the turning that we don't take.

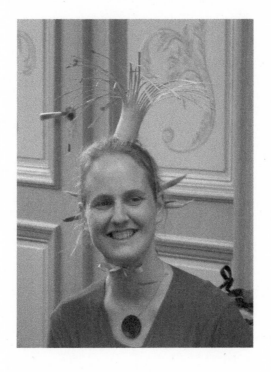

XVII

Sometimes the light at the end of the tunnel
is an oncoming train.

Charles Barkley

And then that Sunday morning. Late June 2009. Nearly five years ago now but I still feel the stinging slap of shock. And I'm still trying to believe the words I first heard then. It was three weeks after the fourth anniversary of Laura's death, the morning after Thomas's seventh birthday party.

Just before the party, doing everything too fast, fumbling and frantic, I sprain my ankle, then later damage the car by reversing into a barrier. Looking back now, I ask myself was there some strange metallic atmosphere in the air? An unidentified ringing sound like a distant alarm bell? Certainly the day begins quite normally. I go to the local Quaker Meeting House in Nailsworth, return home to get the lunch. Then Stephen comes down from his office and tells me that, while I was out, Matthew called from Hereford Hospital. He said – Joslin has cancer and she's dying. There is nothing they can do. It isn't clear yet whether they might be able to save the baby.

I stagger out of the front door, climb the steps onto the steep lawn that edges the drive. My knees fold up and I lie in the grass, howling. In my head, I am hastily doing the sums. Joslin's baby has been in the womb twenty-four weeks. As Laura was. My mind refuses to move further than this.

The grass of the lawn presses against my face. The sky above is entirely innocent. I can't measure the dimensions of this new world. But still the lunch has to be made and so I go in and finish preparing it. Thomas knows that something is wrong so I tell him that Joslin is ill but don't let him know the full details. After Thomas has eaten lunch and left the room I say to Stephen – I know you think I only ever make friends with people with problems. But you can't say I chose this. I couldn't possibly have known.

215

I know, Stephen says. I know.

It isn't fair. Why does this have to land in our lives? Haven't we done our fair share of tragedy? When will it be enough?

I'm not a saint, I'm not even averagely good. I felt like walking away, simply pretending that Joslin and I had never really been friends. But there was no way I could. She was there for me when I needed her and so I would have to be there for her. I would do that for Laura. It was the promise I made to her. *No one else who is grieving or in pain is going to be left to struggle alone if I can do anything to help them.*

But what do you say to someone with young children who is dying aged thirty-five? Someone who is pregnant but knows that the baby might die? I know that I mustn't give myself any time to think, so hastily I call Joslin's mobile. She is calm, friendly.

So I'll see your five Dead Babies, she says. And I'll raise you terminal cancer.

I laugh when I should be wailing because I don't believe any of this is happening. Perhaps if we all keep telling jokes then this will all simply evaporate. I know that I mustn't howl down the phone. Joslin doesn't want that and it won't help. She tells me that the baby is a girl and that she has decided to name her Lily but she says nothing about Lily's chances of survival and I don't ask.

She is too exhausted to talk for long, too shocked and confused. So many doctors and drugs. I ask if I can visit but she doesn't want that. I promise to call again soon. After she's put the phone down, I realise that I'm waiting for the grown-ups to arrive and sort this out. But we are the grown-ups now.

The next few days are a tangle of phone calls and e-mails from concerned friends. Initially it seems that Joslin might only have days to live, that it might be necessary to deliver the baby straightaway, meaning that she will be badly premature and might not survive.

But then the news is slightly better. Joslin might have months to live, maybe even two years. The hospital will delay treating her and leave the baby in the womb until thirty-four weeks. Joslin will be moved to Cheltenham Hospital as they have the best Oncology Centre in the area.

I'm suddenly back in touch with friends at the Meeting House in Brussels. They all want to do something to help but they're too far away. All of them take the news head on. But other Brussels friends react in strange ways, tell me Joslin is definitely going to live. It's just a question of finding the right drugs.

Joslin calls me before the ambulance comes to take her to Cheltenham. The cancer has cracked her spine so she is unable to move. She will never move properly again. She's dreading the journey because even the slightest jolt is agony.

News comes that she's arrived in Cheltenham safely but is too ill for anyone to visit. Friends in Brussels tell me what a relief it is that she is now only fourteen miles from me so I'll be able to go and visit her on their behalf. I feel inadequate and isolated, frightened.

No one in my new life knows Joslin so I can't talk to them about her. On my brisk, smiling school run people don't seem to be involved in messy stuff to do with life and death, or if they are, they don't talk about it. If I mention what's happened, it will surely be viewed as some sort of failing on my part. Or perhaps disasters like this are infectious? Best to steer clear.

I say to myself – Remember, this isn't Zimbabwe, or the

Horn of Africa. But that mantra is failing me now because there is something medieval, Biblical even, in the scale of this. Perhaps it is not surprising that many people have simply decided to alter the story. I have a sense that Someone Out There is trying to bring me down. But I'm not going down. I don't know much – but I know that.

I get a text from Joslin saying that she's allowed visitors. I gather my courage and set off for Cheltenham Hospital. The circus-ballerina woman floating above the earth in the red swirling dress – that woman has died already. Instead Joslin is a twisted lump of flesh, her face the colour of putty. She lies half covered by one of those inadequate green hospital gowns. One of her breasts is visible, the top of a thigh.

It's clear that she's far beyond caring. But I hate to see her like this and find a nurse, insist that more sheets are provided so that she's properly covered up. As I arrange the fresh sheets, my hand brushes against the bump of her pregnancy and a vertigo feeling of sickness washes against me like a wave breaking on a beach.

I'm glad that Joslin at least has a room of her own. It's on the ground floor and has French windows. These only open onto an alleyway but still the breath of fresh air that moves the long net curtains is welcome. I move my chair closer to that window, concentrate on breathing.

Joslin tells me how it all started.

Everyone kept telling me it was just the pregnancy, she says. Then finally they did an MRI scan, found cracks in my spine. No one has cracks in their spine unless they've had a serious accident. So that's when they knew.

The cancer started in her breast but it wasn't detected be-cause of the baby. Pregnancy is a time when everything grows quickly – babies and tumours. By the time that scan was done, the cancer had already spread all over her body. Joslin hasn't seen Ellie and James for several days. She dreads seeing them because they will want to hug her and that will cause her too much pain. She knows there are practical matters that she must address. The custody of the children, her divorce, making a will – but she's too ill to think of any of that.

A nurse from the Maternity Unit arrives to check for the baby's heartbeat.

Go, you must go, Joslin says. Get a coffee and I'll text you when it's safe to come back. I am grateful to her and head over to the canteen, spill scalding coffee on my hand, hear my teeth chatter against the rim of the cup.

I keep seeing an image of Joslin as she was in Brussels, at the Meeting House, when we all made hats out of newspaper and cardboard from the recycling box. I can't remember now why we ever did that – but I do know that everyone else, myself included, made a squashed object out of screwed-up newspaper or a crown out of a cereal box. But Joslin took hold of a cardboard tube and instantly produced a hat that made her look smart enough for Royal Ascot. We were all entranced but she only laughed, shrugged.

Now when I go back to Joslin's room, she asks me about my life and I tell her that I feel under pressure to consider IVF using a donor egg. She tells me that the doctors have told her that the treatment for the cancer will destroy her fertility. As she says this, she starts to cry. I find it strange that she should mourn her fertility when she's losing her life. But perhaps the loss she's facing is so great that she can only grasp a fragment of it.

It all seems so normal, I say. You and I talking like this. But then this door opens in my mind and what I see is so unbelievably terrible that I have to bang the door shut again.

I know, Joslin says. But I must keep easing the door open. The nurses keep trying to give me sleeping pills but this is my journey and I want to be here for it.

A nurse comes in, brings a form to fill in, disappears.

I just want you to understand, I say. The fact that I'm sitting here talking about everyday stuff doesn't mean I haven't seen. And just because I'm not lying on the floor howling in anger and pain, don't think I don't feel like doing that. But me talking about how bad I feel isn't going to help you.

Thanks, she says. You're right. I don't need your pain as well as mine.

As I leave, she says – What I've got to think is that it doesn't really matter whether you've got two days, or two years, or two decades. It's still about how you want to live those days. I don't want the days I have – no matter how few or how many – eaten up in bitterness and grief.

Part of her reaction may be shock and drugs – but much of it is plain old-fashioned courage.

I know the drill now. I recognise the liberating euphoria which shock brings. I must make the best of these moments of energy, courage, acceptance. They will not last. And anyway I am the lucky one. I will walk out of this alive. Joslin will not, her baby may not.

I go back to the hospital regularly over the next few weeks. One of my plays is being rehearsed at the Everyman Theatre, which is only a few streets from the hospital, so I go and see a rehearsal and then go on to the hospital. These two worlds can be hard to balance – the luminous, laughing, living girls who act in the play and the grey, limping, hairless patients I see in the corridors of the Oncology Centre.

I am going through a crash course in how you deal with the

terminally ill. It's all about what people want to know, and what they don't want to know, at any given time. It can be hard to keep up, not to hit the wrong note.

Sometimes Joslin is absolutely clear about what is happening. But at other times she is furious because a nurse or a friend has mentioned death. She's still got years to live, she says. Many people last far longer than expected, she'll be home with the children soon. How dare people drag her down with their negativity?

At the hospital I manage bedpans, help Joslin put on deodorant, hold bowls while she throws up, again and again. I didn't know I would be able to do these things. I do not consider myself courageous. Courage implies choice and I'm not aware of any choice.

One day I arrive and Joslin is in agony, clutching her head. I don't understand why they can't give her more painkillers. I always thought that in the modern world people don't have to endure horrible levels of pain. But this is wrong.

A nurse explains to me that the cancer may have gone to Joslin's brain. Tests have been done and the results will arrive by the end of the day. Wayland and Matthew arrive from Hay-on-Wye. They are here often but I have not seen them much as we try to spread our visits out, make sure she isn't alone too much.

For that unending day, we ride the storms of Joslin's pain and anger, waiting always for the next wave to break. Occasionally we sit out in the alleyway, on the concrete steps. Above, a narrow strip of August sky is white, motionless. Shouts or cheers rise up from the cricket festival in the grounds of Cheltenham College. I have never smoked but wonder if I should take it up.

Finally the results of the tests arrive. Wayland stays with Joslin while she talks to the doctor, and I sit out on the steps, staring at the ground. Mercifully it seems that the cancer hasn't spread to her brain. A wave carries us forward into gasping relief. But this only means that Joslin and the baby have a little more time.

For a long while, I am too tired to get up from the steps. Wayland and Matthew are with Joslin and I can hear their distant voices. The light is fading, the air chills. My bones are stiff, my head rests against the wall. Matthew brings me some strong, burnt-tasting coffee from a machine and, finally, I am able to stand up, head for home.

I buy Joslin silly, luxurious presents. I know that other people disapprove of this. Joslin is not a materialistic person and now she needs to address her spiritual journey, put her worldly affairs in order. I don't give a damn. I just want her to have five minutes of pleasure and if a present will do that then I'll buy any number of them.

But buying gifts for the terminally ill can be complicated. I know that Joslin likes a certain range of organic, herbal face creams but I can't work out from the website which cream will be best for her so I ring the company.

Our anti-ageing creams are very popular, the voice on the phone says.

Oh yes, good idea.

And then I think again. How incredibly tactless to buy anti-ageing creams for someone who is dying. Joslin would probably see the humour but still I choose another product and am left considering what a luxury it is to grow old.

I go to the hospital and, just as I'm leaving, I meet Joslin's consultant. I struggle to remember now exactly what happened. Did he say that he needed to talk to Joslin? Did he ask me if it might be possible for me to stay a while?

Something about that brief encounter – my mind goes into rebellion if I try to think of it. All I know is that I need to get out of the hospital, that I can't stay longer. I do have to pick up Thomas from school but I only use that as an excuse. I have to leave, to run, to stop the dizzy panic, the sickness, the screaming inside.

I go back to the car, start driving along the A46 out of Cheltenham. Then I'm drowning, water in my mouth and lungs, pulling me under. I know with a terrible certainty that the consultant was going to deliver bad news. And it was about the baby.

I pull into a car park. Is that place something to do with an insurance company? Or a hotel? Certainly it is corporate, clean, well organised. Steep hills, stippled grey and green, are rising in the distance, road junctions are knotted everywhere with cars dashing past, narrowly missing each other. Brakes scream, everything smells of petrol. The world tips and I start to scream and I can't stop because I know with absolute certainty that Joslin's baby would die. I scream until my lungs ache and I can't stop coughing.

Then finally I get out of the car, lie on a stretch of grass between parked cars, listened to the traffic. Eventually I get up, prop myself against the car, call one of the mums at school and ask her to pick up Thomas. Then I call my mum. I don't tell her what has happened but listen to her talking about normal things.

A litter of puppies, the weather. Such a lovely walk down the fields. And she'd called her brothers in Lincolnshire. All the family news. Still listening, I look around me, up to the blurring hills and see that evening is coming, the shadows spilling and I am cold and stiff, dirty from sitting against the wheel of the car. I say goodbye to Mum and get up. No call came from the hospital. No bad news. It was all something I had imagined.

Increasingly I am unable to breathe. I really don't want to go to the doctor but finally I'm left with no choice. I am diagnosed as having Post Traumatic Stress Disorder. The doctor tells me that the problem is not just Laura's death. It's the fact that the miscarriages keep taking me back to what happened, and now the risk to baby Lily is doing the same. The wound is never given the chance to heal.

Initially I am rather pleased with the diagnosis. It always helps to have a big name for something. And surely nothing can be expected of anyone with such a dire condition? Finally Matron will be convinced. I'm not just skiving, malingering, failing to pull myself together. I hope that I might be moving closer to the moment when I will crouch in a corner, babbling and dribbling. But nothing changes.

I consider trying the words out on a few people but the whole thing sounds too grandiose. Surely PTSD is Vietnam, Iraq, Afghanistan? But I do begin to read about trauma and what I read makes me feel less alone. People who return from war zones can't adapt to normal life. They have seen something so terrible that they can't understand how other people are continuing with their merry little lives.

They live cut off, isolated, unable to go out and talk to people. They feel that they simply are not occupying the same world as those around them. All of that makes sense to me. Then I read about the cure for PTSD and there isn't one.

Plans are made for the day when Joslin's baby will be delivered. Joslin and other friends ask me if I'll be there. They have no idea of the magnitude of what they are asking. I mention to my doctor that I feel the need to do this.

She is adamant – no, absolutely not. Not under any circumstances. I know she's right. And this isn't a purely selfish decision. What Joslin needs is someone calm and able to focus on her needs. She doesn't need me collapsing in a heap. But it's hard to tell her that I won't be there. Finally Matthew kindly does that for me.

Friends in Brussels raise money so that a homeopath whom Joslin trusts can come over from where she now lives in Ireland to be with Joslin at the birth. I take care not even to ask when exactly the birth will take place. When a text arrives from Wayland saying that the baby has been safely delivered my lungs are suddenly able to contain more air.

XVIII

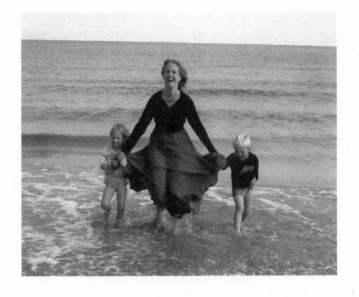

Living well is the best revenge.

George Herbert

When I was a child I spent a lot of my time watching middle-aged women. I wanted to know what the future might hold. My mum was not part of this study as I knew her to be unique, her own creation. She wore men's trousers, cut off at the knee and made into plus fours. Her hands were crusted red, her hair an electric shock, her pockets full of nails and binder twine. Her only make-up was a cracked tube of pink Max Factor which lived in the glove pocket of the car.

She was a person I could admire but not a model I could replicate. But the other mothers? Brittle and raw, they kept themselves and everything around them locked down tight. Their mouths turned down. They shrugged, sighed, raised their eyebrows, uttered short and strangled sentences through locked jaws. It was clear they had been cheated of something but I didn't know what.

The worst were the ones with blonde helmet haircuts, carefully tended waists, expensive tans, tasteful gold jewellery, suede boots. All of this assembled and maintained with such painful care that surely it could compensate for whatever they had lost? And yet it clearly failed to do so.

I was certain of one thing – I was not going to finish up as one of those women. No chance that I would be left at home sweeping the hearth. I was going to the ball and I didn't care what I might have to do to get there. Lying, cheating, numerous small acts of selfishness – all would be acceptable in order to rise above the fate that had clearly engulfed those school-run mums.

But now I look in the mirror and think that I – with my oh-so-tasteful clothes – am fast becoming one of those women. Increasingly I am settling for those same cheap compensations – good clothes, a stylish haircut. *I have no choice about the*

Dead Babies but I don't have to be fat and badly dressed.
  Somewhere there must be another route but I can't find it.
And now, when I look in the mirror, my mouth has a clamped
look and I find myself giving a brittle shrug. I even buy some
waterproof mascara. It does have many benefits in difficult
times.

Baby Lily needs specialist care and so she and Joslin are
moved from the Oncology Centre to the Neonatal Unit. When
I go to visit, I walk the same corridors I walked when I had my
last miscarriage. Had that baby lived, I would now be coming
to the hospital to give birth. I dread the Neonatal Unit. The
thought of seeing a premature baby brings sweat blooming to
my skin. But I never reach the door of the unit. Joslin, in a
wheelchair, is waiting for me in the corridor.
  Get me out of here. Now.
  I catch hold of the wheelchair, spin it around.
  Quick, she says, before anyone sees.
  I speed the wheelchair into the lift. At the main reception, a
nurse tries to question me but I wave at her merrily, shove the
wheelchair out of the door. Outside, in the August sun, Joslin
and I stop and laugh.
  Like breaking out of jail, she says, and puts her head back
to feel the sun.
  We head towards the Bath Road. If the wheelchair jolts
even slightly then Joslin is in terrible pain. We get coffee and
sandwiches and head for the lawns outside Cheltenham
College. Joslin eases herself down so she can sit on the grass.
We eat our sandwiches, drink coffee. For Joslin, even these
simple pleasures seem miraculous. She tells me about baby
Lily, the children, her plans for when she finally gets home.
She's going to get a van which can take her wheelchair and

which has beds as well. Then set off round the world. She's been searching the web, planning where she wants to go.

She's also found a clinic in Santa Fe, New Mexico, that regularly cures people with terminal cancer. Perhaps she could stop off there on her world trip?

It's hard to know how to react to this. Is it positive that she's considering all the options? Or is she deluded? I know that many of Joslin's friends tend to the latter view. I prefer to allow myself to be caught up in the dream – but soon the conversation darkens.

I want to talk about death, she says. About what happens, whether there is anything afterwards. No one talks to me about those things but I know you will.

OK, I say. Yes. Of course.

Of course, I've always believed there is nothing, Joslin says.

Even nothing must be something, I say.

Do you really think so?

Yes. But I don't know what.

For a long time we talk, sitting out on the grass, turning the question over.

What I reckon, Joslin says, is that, when you die, your spirit breaks up into many different pieces. Parts of it may finish up in places far and near. In your children and friends. Or perhaps dispersed into the atmosphere, turning into the leaves of a tree, or being washed away in a stream. What do you reckon?

Yes, I say. Yes.

I am taking the conversation seriously but I'm also gauging what Joslin needs.

Compost, she says. I've always reckoned I'll make damn good compost.

We dream of the flowers and vegetables which will grow in Joslin compost. And then we talk of a photograph that she has on the hospital wall. It was taken before she got ill and shows her with Ellie and James, on the Isle of Tiree, which is part of the Inner Hebrides. The three of them are there, on the beach, hand in hand, running in the waves.

Then I admit that I've been wondering if, when Joslin becomes compost, she'll meet Laura. And I describe a ridiculous sentimental image which keeps appearing in my mind – Joslin like the Virgin Mary, eyes raised to heaven, with Laura in her arms. We both laugh but we also agree that, right now, any image will do.

My life stumbles on. I put the washing machine on, hang clothes on the line, load the dishwasher, start work on an interesting theatre commission, tell Thomas to switch the Harry Potter DVD off. Now. No, listen to what I'm saying. Right now.

The building work at the house hasn't even started yet and we can't get in touch with the adoption agency again until it is finished. I know anyway that we're never going to adopt. I need to focus on Thomas now. He is easily enough for me and he grows more lovely, funnier, every day. I mustn't lose what I have while searching for what I don't have.

The days are hard but at least we know where we are now. At least there is no hope. But still people send me articles about a new doctor, a new treatment. The press is full of reports about a grandmother in her sixties in Romania who has had a baby, or a woman who doesn't have a uterus who is pregnant. My mother doesn't understand why I won't try donor eggs. My sister generously offers to donate eggs.

I can give up – but other people cannot.

Giving up? To me, it's like the sticking plaster question when you're a child. A fall in the playground, a plaster applied to the cut knee. But then the day arrives when the plaster has to be removed. One of my friends is a coward. She won't let her mother just rip the plaster off. Instead she spends days peeling it slowly, doubtless feeling hair after hair pulled, prickling, from her knee. I can't understand this. I say to my mother – Pull it as hard as you can so it comes off really quickly. I prefer my pain short and sharp.

I attend the stillbirth support group often now. There you see all the great circus of grief. People who are not just naked but who have had their skin peeled away from their bones. All the normal rules of social interaction evaporate. Pain spills everywhere, burns on the tongue, closes the throat. The very air of the room buzzes with loss.

People behave in extraordinary ways. One man has to be politely asked to go out into the hall after he has spent quarter of an hour making business calls loudly on his mobile phone. Another man – an electrician by profession – becomes obsessed by a flickering light, finds a ladder, examines the fuse box, interrupts the grieving parents below with regular updates from the ladder top on the problems which doubtless exist with the wiring in the building.

Occasionally there are moments of mad humour, as when a woman arrives clutching a baby blanket and says to the group – On the anniversary of my son's death, my husband jumped out of a plane.

This news hits the room with a dull crash – we are ready for stillbirth but not suicide. Everyone gasps, someone sobs. The woman speaking looks confused.

Oh no, she says. No. I didn't mean that. No. You see. He jumped out wearing a parachute. To raise money for charity.

At this group, I don't speak because my own story has become too big to tell. And also because bitter experience has already revealed to me that my brand of grief – which involves a sizeable measure of flippancy – is not to most people's taste. Grief, like everything else, has its rules. Encounters with The Grief Police can be bruising. It is best not to stray too far from the litany of lambs and angels and light.

But I do listen and offer whatever comfort I can. *No one else who is grieving or in pain is going to be left to struggle alone if I can do anything to help them.* One woman says to me – What I'm doing is trying to identify something from before. Some part of my life that I can still recognise from before our baby died.

I consider this statement. Is it too extreme? Sadly I don't think it is.

Often women come who have suffered a stillbirth but now have another baby. They find themselves surrounded by caring relatives who are furiously celebrating, determined to put the past behind them. But the mothers themselves are often distressed, confused. Some of them reject the new baby entirely. One woman says to me again and again – I can't touch him, I can't look at him. He's the wrong baby. The wrong baby.

But what shocks me more than anything are the medical negligence deaths. Every week couples turn up with stories of hospital incompetence that are initially hard to believe – but which become horribly repetitive and familiar. I've known for a long time that the UK is recorded as number thirty-four out of thirty-five in a table which measures rates of stillbirth in countries with comparable living standards.

But it is only now that I meet the victims that I fully understand what this means. I've always accepted that I had to go through what I went through. It was just bad luck. But the discovery that there are others who have suffered the same due to incompetence whips me into a rage.

I do endless research, speak to women whose babies have been lost because of medical negligence, the lawyers who represent them. Generally these women get a payout of £10,000. Most of them say – I could just about cope. Until the moment when I realised that exactly the same thing had happened to another woman in the same hospital just the week after our baby died. That's what broke me.

Could this question of medical negligence become the end to my own story? *So very sad what happened to her – but then she became this amazing campaigner for safe maternity care.* I would like to be that campaigning person, using my own grief to insist on safety for others, but I haven't the energy or the courage any more.

The builders move into our house. The drive is crammed with vans, a site office is established in the cellar. The scaffolding goes up. The garden turns into a ploughed field. Initially I enjoy the builders. They break into our solitude, have no considerations beyond the practical. Untypical builders, they are unfailingly polite and helpful. Our site manager is called Pete Jobbins – he's short and solid, with silver hair and remains positive, no matter what.

Every day he arrives at eight, with a team of men, gripping cigarettes and flasks of tea, joking as they come down the drive. Sometimes as many as ten arrive and we see teams of them, silhouetted against the sky, working on the chimneys, the guttering, the stonework, the roof.

Every inch of the house is covered with that thick, dry builder's dust which sticks to hair, clothes, the back of the throat. Someone forgets that the bath isn't plumbed in and turns on a tap upstairs. Water floods into the hall. Peter Jobbins gets stuck in a water tank and for a while it looks as though the fire brigade might have to be called. A man slices into an artery on his wrist while working on the roof and has to be taken to Casualty. Blood stains the doorstep and trails up the drive.

At lunchtime, the house smells of takeaway curries. The builders read *The Sun*, crumpling it between their dusty fingers.

Here, have you seen this one? This bird's in court asking for compensation because her boss told her she's got lovely tits. I mean, would you credit it? What is her problem?

One day I pick Thomas up from school and he has had a bad day. I should comfort him but I've had a bad day as well and have nothing left to give him. We walk back to the car together and suddenly I have an idea. Listen, I say. You're feeling angry and I'm feeling angry so we're going to break the rules, do something you're not normally allowed to do.

What?

When we get in the car, you can swear all the way home. You can use any word you want and you can shout it as loud as you want. What do you reckon?

We drive out of the school gates and I wind down the windows. I start and he quickly joins me. Bugger. Fuck. Wanker. Prat.

Our voices get louder and louder as we cross the Common. Tit. Bastard. Bloody.

We are screaming at the top of our voices, filth tumbling out. Bollocks. Bloody. Bloody. Fuck.

As the car stops in the drive, Thomas shouts – More, more. Please more.

No. That's it. Just once every six months on the drive home. That's all.

But we feel so much better that we often wind the windows down, yell abuse at no one, enjoy the laughter afterwards, the sense of release and euphoria. I make Thomas promise not to repeat the words at school – but I know he will.

Winter closes in on us. The days are grey and silent, the skies soft with gathering snow. The water is switched off, the lights fuse continually. We all wear three jumpers, gloves, scarves, thermal leggings. One night, when the power and gas are off, the three of us sit on Stephen's and my bed – an island of comfort amidst bare, dusty boards, drying plaster and stacked furniture. We eat takeaway pizza and, as soon as we've finished, we all get into bed to keep warm and drift towards sleep, still wearing our clothes, pressed together for warmth.

As the year sinks towards its bitter end, we are gradually defeated. One day I arrive back from teaching in Oxford and am greeted by an evil smell which seems to spread right across the Stroud Valleys. A drain which has clearly been blocked for years is in the process of being unblocked. I step over piles of boards in the hall, head for the telephone. I need a hot bath, a proper meal, a warm bed. I ring a hotel which is just across the Common from us and book us in for the weekend. When Stephen and Thomas return they agree that this is a good idea.

Our dinner at the hotel feels amazingly luxurious. We talk about the wonders of the night ahead which will be spent in a warm bed. But just as we are walking back to the room the hotel manager waylays us, wringing his hands. They've had a problem with the boiler, someone has been called. But. But. We head back to the room, shaking our heads, laughing.

Thomas puts on a James Bond DVD. I sit down at the dressing table, stare at myself in the mirror. Ah well, at least my hair looks good.

One morning, driving across the Common, after dropping Thomas at school, I stop the car in the National Trust car park, prop myself against the bonnet, take a few deep breaths. The temperature is below freezing, the day is stationary, placid, the light subdued. The views have no depth to them, their colours merge. A thought comes to me with sudden force – *In all of this I have reckoned without the force of the human will.*

In our generation, the human will is unfashionable. Everybody has to be allowed to feel what they feel, express, process. The worst thing you can say to the suffering is – Pull yourself together.

Certainly in my twenties and thirties, I ascribed to the view that emotional authenticity is everything. But now I begin to realise that there may be events too big to process. Sometimes the only way to survive is to get up and walk on without looking back. The human will is incredibly strong, capable of anything. And pretending isn't necessarily wrong. It can be understood as rehearsing.

I start to understand my mother and my long-departed grandmother in a way I never have before. They were wartime women with English stiff upper lips. Busy, practical, efficient, they smiled no matter what. Ten years ago – having read the psychotherapy textbooks – I would have accused them of denial. Now I understand that sometimes it is better to smile and pretend it never happened. As a woman, you do eventually turn into your mother, but by the time that happens, you have forgiven her.

As I drive home along the top lane, I meet those sinister single magpies, still hopping and flapping malevolently. But I'm not frightened of them any more. Instead I wind down the window and shout at them – Bring it on, you buggers. I'm ready.

XIX

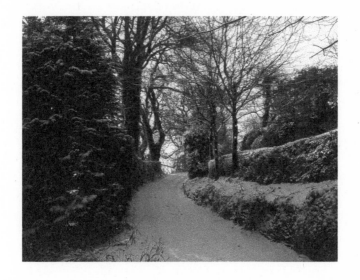

What a wonderful life I've had!
I only wish I'd realised it sooner.

Colette

I am haunted by babies, dead, unborn and unclaimed. They live in a dark winter forest of silver birch trees, where the tree trunks, branchless, glisten in the moonlight. And between those trees the babies move, like sprites. Seen and unseen, dancing with arms and hands outstretched, their intricate feet leaving no prints.

There are so many of them. The miscarried babies, the Russian and Chinese babies we didn't adopt, the IVF babies who were never more than two or three cells, invisible to the naked eye, but who play in the forest all the same, their distant laughter receding as they spin and twist deeper and deeper into the skeletal trees.

I long to walk through the forest, to stretch out my hands to them, to gather them all to me, to feel their laughter bubbling, the touch of their tiny, damp hands in mine. But the forest is closed to me. Every time I try to enter, it dissolves. And every time I stretch out my hand to those babies, they dance away from me, laughing, and are lost amidst the trees. Shadows are harder to battle than armies. They have no shape, every time I lunge for them they dissolve.

The question which troubles me is this: maybe what happened to me is normal? Maybe I just didn't understand. Certainly by the time you're forty, something nasty will have happened to you, or to someone you love. So what level of tragedy should one expect in the course of a human life? Certainly everyone I meet now has suffered some terrible loss. But are these people typical? Or has my bad luck magnet attracted them? And are there others out there still in the non-tragedy world? Or does that world simply not exist?

And if everybody is in Tragedy-ville, to one degree or another, then why doesn't it show on their faces? Are they simply deciding not to let it show? And is that decision made out of generosity to others? Out of a desire not to involve others in their worry? Or is it a mass denial that damages us all?

Whatever the answer, I am determined to find a way out of Tragedy-ville. I have ripped the sticking plaster off with a flick of my wrist and ignored the hair-stripped pain it leaves behind. Time to move on, to start again. We need an end to the story, a new beginning. But the new route I'm looking for still doesn't appear.

And then late one night, in a New York bar, Stephen tells our story to an American colleague. You need a surrogate mom. That's what we do in the States. Why not?

Stephen arrives back from his trip, tries the idea out on me. It's evening and I'm carrying a basket of washing upstairs. The last thing I need is hope. We've been through all this before. Why doesn't he understand?

No, I say. No, no, no, no, no. Surrogate mothers live in trailer parks in America, and they smoke and drink throughout the pregnancy. Then everyone finishes up in court – or on a reality TV show.

But then I look down from the turn in the stairs and see the disappointment on Stephen's face. He needs some thread of hope, no matter how fragile. The laundry basket feels like it's full of rocks. Our marriage is a fabric that has been mended too often. Soon it will tear in our hands, flake away into rags. I need to get us through another month or two.

I'll look into it, I say. See what I can find out.

It's winter and Stephen is away often. With the builders in the house I can't write. Do you want this socket here? Or here? Was it linen white or porcelain white? Ah yes, there does appear to be water pouring down the wall. Yes, I'll get it switched off at the mains. But we'll have to put the electrics off as well.

I find myself a studio outside the house to work. It is a bubble of warmth and quiet. I switch off my mobile and continue to work on my novel and on a new play. I am the least prolific of writers and never actually finish anything, but strangely I know that I'm writing better now. As I have ceased to exist myself, I find it easy to enter into other worlds.

Later I pick Thomas up from school, light the wood burner and make him a cheesy toasty, and then we curl up together on the sofa, amidst the dust and boxes full of floor tiles. Thomas has discovered computers and is obsessed by a website called Club Penguin. On this site he can acquire virtual penguins, furnish an igloo, go on fishing trips and take his penguins out for pizza.

After Thomas has gone to bed, I read surrogacy stories. I tell myself that I am doing this for Stephen but the truth is that I am less good at ripping-the-plaster-off-quickly than I pretend to be. And this research is harmless, isn't it? Just Club Penguin for adults really. I find an article about a surrogate mother who is an artist. A photograph shows her in front of an easel, pregnant, blondely blurred with a distant, secretive smile. Could she have a child for me? I remind myself that this woman is probably featured in a magazine precisely because she is untypical of her breed.

I discover that there are two kinds of surrogacy: traditional surrogacy, which is when a woman has a baby for you, and gestational surrogacy which is when a woman is implanted with your egg, or some other egg, and carries that baby for you, despite the fact that she has no genetic link to that baby. Technology has only recently made the latter possible. In the *Daily Mail*, gestational surrogacy is referred to as 'rent a womb', and reports suggest that in India, the Ukraine or Kazakhstan it costs only £8,000.

One evening Stephen comes back from London with a copy of the Evening Standard. On the front page is an article about a case in the High Court concerning a couple who have won the right to bring surrogate twins back to England from India. We both read the article several times but then agree that surrogacy in a developing country isn't an option. The income disparities are too great, the possibilities for exploitation too real. We don't want a child if that will involve a risk to another woman's health or happiness.

But maybe America is different? No one there needs to become a surrogate mum for financial reasons, do they? We are unsure about that. There is no social security there, is there? Although we have these discussions, they are just a way of passing the time. A way for me to offer Stephen some hope. Surrogacy is immoral, exploitative. We have given up, definitely and completely.

Joslin never makes it to the clinic in Santa Fe but finishes up in a semi-detached house in Bromsgrove, with a group of other cancer patients, being fed evil-tasting herbal brews by a New Age witch. She is the rebel in this group, the one who questions. Others don't like this. She rings me sounding disappointed, depressed.

Surely drinking something which tastes quite this bad can't possibly be good for me? she says. It's the same with all these support group situations, she continues. The other people have got cancer, of course. But none of them are terminal. And so, when they meet me their faces brighten, their bodies start to come back to life because they remember that it could be worse. And that's great for them. Lovely. But for me? What is there for me? I would like a role beyond being the person who reminds others that it could be worse.

I would not insult Joslin by comparing her situation to mine. But I know what she's talking about. Because at the stillbirth support groups, I also play the role of the person who reminds everyone that it could be worse.

And yet I continue to go to that group and find it enlightening, strangely comforting. One evening a man turns up – a blokey guy in a denim jacket, trainers, a crew cut and an earring. He's overweight, has full red cheeks, an open, grinning face. The words fall from him in a manic, spitting rush.

He had a great little butt my son, he says. That's how we knew he was mine.

He says this with a raucous laugh, rubs his meaty hands together, continues to tell his story, like a man rehearsing a stand-up comedy routine.

The same big arse we've all got in our family and the same big nose. A great little guy. Only two weeks ago, since he was born.

With a sickening jolt, the group understands that this man doesn't know fully that his son is dead. His voice runs on. All a good joke down the pub. I feel the others around me wince, their flesh creeping away, but their eyes remain staunchly fixed on him, letting him know he is heard.

This is the miracle of the support group – the way in which, without even making eye contact, this group of people around him know what to do. No one tries to jolt him into reality. Instead they chuckle a little and smile, ask affectionate questions. What was his weight? Did he have much hair? Ooh, lovely. Do you have any photos? They understand that this man is a man in deep shock. And this is the only vocabulary he has.

Cheeky little bugger, he was. And a bit fat, just like me. Called him Sean. Wife and I have always liked that name. Got it on the door of his room all ready.

Around him people nod and sigh. How lovely to have his name on the door. And I sit there with them, humbled. Because somehow this group of random, unexceptional people, unexpectedly thrown into a pit of horror, are able to behave with generosity, dignity, compassion. Are able to weave this joyous, shattered man into their web of comfort. The truth is that our own pain is not what will destroy us but imagining the pain of others.

I go to meet Joslin at the hospital where she's having chemotherapy. The treatment room is strangely like a hairdresser's with people sitting in chairs against the walls, plugged into machines. Except that most of the people at this hairdresser's don't have any hair.

The machines make a cheerful bing-bing-bing noise when the infusions are finished. Relatives sit on two rows of chairs in the centre, back to back, like a game of musical chairs. Most of the patients wear sweat pants and T-shirts but Joslin and I sit next to a woman who wears a sharp black suit, pinched in around her tiny waist, towering red high heels on the end of spaghetti legs.

Her name is June. Her blonde hair is neatly blow-dried, sweeps elegantly back from her face. She burns with a luminous good health. Her smile is charming, warm. She has read every book about cancer and she knows everything about alternative therapies, special diets, acupuncture.

A doctor in Germany has had remarkable results using linseed oil and cottage cheese. The Santa Fe clinic isn't all it's cracked up to be. Some people rate the witch in Bromsgrove but others suspect her brews are only drain water. June pats her shining curls as she talks but leans forward to whisper – It's a wig, of course.

We agree that it's extraordinarily convincing. June promises to give Joslin the details of the company that supplied the wig. I like June and am pleased when she and Joslin swap phone numbers. But too soon Joslin is called to see the consultant and June's treatment is at an end.

As I'm sitting outside the consultant's room, waiting, June sashays past, says how much she enjoyed talking to us. Of course, she says. None of that stuff – the diets and all that. Makes no difference. But you need to take control, to feel like you're doing something. Fighting. That's what's important. And with that she sets off down the corridor on her elegant heels, turns back to give me a bright little wave.

A woman in her fifties turns up at the stillbirth support group. She's wearing a shapely business suit and her brown hair is neatly blow-dried but her eyes are pink and swollen. She says – I just don't get it. I don't understand. It's twenty-five years ago now. And I'm listening to the radio and someone is talking about a stillbirth and I'm ambushed – completely. Back there again. When is it ever going to be finished? When am I finally going to get closure on this?

Closure. The word lands dully in the room. So often people turn up here wanting closure. I don't believe it exists and I suspect that quite a number of the other members of this group don't believe in it either. We've seen the women in their eighties who haven't got closure. I take care what I say, but I can't help thinking that the quest for closure is nothing more than another burden which modern psycho-babble has laid at the door of the grieving.

Now that the builders have gone I set about de-cluttering the house again. That's the word that is used nowadays: de-cluttering. And there are even professional de-clutterers. It seems odd that we should need a whole profession simply to defend us from our own possessions.

I sort and stack and reduce, take more and more things to the charity shop. As I work I sometimes ask myself what I am doing. And the answer comes to me quite clearly. I'm getting ready for death. There is nothing morbid or anxious in this statement. I simply have the feeling that when death comes I want to be ready to catch onto its swirling coat. And I don't want to leave much behind for anyone else to clear up.

I go to the Quaker Meeting House and an elderly man tells a story. It goes like this. A vicar in a rural village goes to call on an old man. They have a cup of tea and the old man then offers to show the vicar his garden. They go out of the back door together and the vicar is thrilled by the tumbling mass of flowers and vegetables, the trees laden with fruit.

And so he turns to the old man and says – So what do you think the Almighty has to do with this?

The old man thinks for a while and then says – Well, vicar, I really can't say. But I would comment that when this place was left to the Almighty, it looked a terrible mess.

The story stays in my head for days afterwards. For me, it's about man and God in cooperation, about finding forces of goodness in the world and aligning yourself with them. And it makes me remember why I became a Quaker and some shred of my lost faith returns. It never did matter whether there is a God or there isn't. It's only about what you do. Just find the forces of goodness in the world – and they are all around the place all day – and align yourself with them. It's really that simple. You don't need to know more.

One night Stephen and I look at American surrogacy websites together. They carry adverts for nail bars in California and wireless hoovers. Stephen flicks to the page about costs. Every possible expense is listed there, including what it will cost if the surrogate gets pregnant with triplets and you want to abort one or more of the foetuses. Which is very precise, at least. Stephen clicks another button labelled financing and it takes us into an entirely different website offering breast reduction, teeth whitening, bald-patch fixing – and infertility treatment.

Great, Stephen says. You get your boobs done, I'll get my teeth whitened and we'll buy a baby. Maybe that way we'll be eligible for some kind of discount.

But then the conversation turns serious and I ask him if he really thinks we could do this.

I don't know, he says. But I think for men surrogacy isn't so complicated. After all, as a man, you're always relying on some woman to have a baby for you.

We move to another website crammed with photographs of soft-focus young women with blissful faces and long blonde hair holding smiling, chubby blue-eyed babies. Welcome to the Palm Springs Center for Surrogacy – Making Happy Endings. Stephen and I snigger but I suspect that he's aware, as I am, that a happy ending is exactly what we need.

Stephen develops asthma. I didn't know that you could start getting asthma in middle age. At night his coughing and wheezing rattles the house. Also his balance is poor and the medical profession don't understand why. I begin to send e-mails to agencies. The replies come back, swift and kind. All of them begin with that American mantra: I'm sorry for your loss. A few years ago I might have found that irritating, but now it seems better than European silence and form-shuffling. All of the American e-mails say yes, yes and yes. For a fee, of course. It's a long time since anyone has said yes to Stephen and me, fee or no fee. God Bless America.

But could we really do this? Surely it is morally wrong? In the evenings, sitting in the kitchen, after I have burnt the supper and Thomas has finally gone to bed, Stephen and I have long conversations about this. I don't like the idea of an anonymous egg donor, even though I know women who have chosen that route. Surely every child has the right to know its genetic heritage? But if you know the woman who donates the eggs, and you tell the resulting child the truth from the beginning, then is that acceptable?

Maybe, because then you could show the child a photo-graph, offer them a meeting. It would be like adoption with-out the rejection. But how do you find someone you know to donate an egg? My sister has offered. Is it more weird to bring up your sister's child? Or to bring up a child to whom you have no genetic link? Answer: it's all weird, very weird. Too weird to take seriously. We are sensible, puritanical English people. When we can't have what we want, we bear our suf-fering nobly. Rip the sticking plaster off quickly and move on.

XX

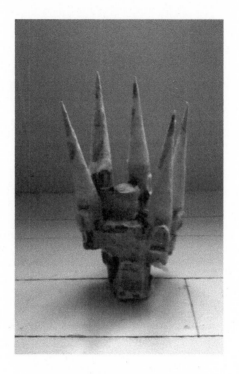

Forgiveness is giving up all hope
of having had a better past.

Anne Lamott

Joslin suggests to me that it might be useful for me to write about Laura's death, the miscarriages. I laugh at this idea. Dear old Joslin, how simplistic she is. For goodness' sake, I am a professional writer, I tell other people's stories. I don't do writing-as-therapy. I make no judgement about others who do, but it's not my thing.

But soon after Joslin makes this suggestion, I find myself sorting through piles of old notebooks and journals. I'm shocked by how much there is. And I remember the person I used to be, the person who recorded the shapes of leaves, the patterns of clouds, the scenes observed from train windows. A person constantly overwhelmed by wonder at what Jack, from the Quaker Meeting House in Brussels, once described as the sheer there-ness of things.

What happened to that person? All these notes and scribblings. A memoir I didn't even know I had written? I start to look through them, remember my friend and his suggested title for any memoir I might write: *The Spectre at the Feast*. How much work would it take to put it all in order? Hours. And anyway, I'm not interested. But then I start to read endless memoirs, trying to understand the form. To me it seems they divide into two types: books written by those who have had amazing experiences but can't write, and books written by people who write like angels but nothing of interest has ever happened to them. I doubt that I would be able to bridge the gap.

But increasingly I am unable to find Joslin's idea laughable. The most obvious ideas are always the most easily overlooked. We all go to the ends of the earth searching for something that we believe to be essential to our happiness, and later find it on our own doorsteps. I buy a new notebook and try out a few words. But I'm not firing on all syllables, and so give up.

I can't sleep at night and the surrogacy websites don't sleep either. I come across an online database of American women who are offering to act as egg donors. On this site you can fill out a form and they'll find you a donor. Height? Hair colour? Ethnicity? Education? Eye colour? Build? I put in my own details. Then I change five foot six to five foot eight and hair colour from brown/blonde to blonde.

The computer whirrs and details come up. There she is: twenty-four years old, tall, with blue eyes and long blonde hair. She speaks several languages and is of German origin, has a Master's degree in music and has decided to donate her eggs to help an infertile couple. Also she needs some money so that she can pursue her cello studies. Other details are supplied: she has long fingers, does voluntary work for disadvantaged children.

Why would I want my child if I could have this woman's child? My fingers are stubby, my French and Spanish are dodgy, I only reached grade five on the piano. The cello-playing woman with the long fingers becomes part of my fantasy. I start to imagine the child that she will give me. This is dangerous, I should stop.

But the surrogacy idea does provide an answer to all our problems. I won't have to get pregnant or give birth. I won't have to go for tests or scans. The child will be Stephen's child. But is any of this legally possible? I search the internet but can find no information about anyone who has brought an American surrogate baby back from the US to England.

Stephen and I discuss again the possibility of using an egg donor. In the past my answer to this has always been a clear 'no'. But now I give the question more thought and realise that, although I am definitely saying no to another pregnancy, to any more medical treatment, the idea of a donor egg doesn't bother me at all. As long as that egg isn't going to be inside me then I'm happy.

But why would we have to use a donor egg? Stephen says. We could use your eggs.

No, I say.

But why not?

Because I'm just not prepared to get involved in any of this unless it has a very high chance of success – and we already know my eggs are no good. And, you know, any clinic would even advise us against taking up my sister's kind offer just because she's thirty-seven and they consider that too old. The statistics just aren't good enough.

Oh right. But don't you mind about not using yours?

No. In all honesty, I don't. Not at all. I suppose I just gave up on the idea that I'd have another child that's genetically related to me a long time back. I would have gone ahead with the adoption idea. I was really ready to do that – so I'm already long past all that genetic stuff. Any baby will do fine for me as long as it's alive. Really.

I can't find anyone who has ever brought a US surrogate baby back into the UK, but I do find a lawyer who specialises in surrogacy and Stephen and I go to visit her. Her name is Natalie Gamble and she works from a business park on the edge of Poole. She is thin and intense with long, black hair. She is calm, professional, clear in her advice. To her, surrogacy isn't weird. Potential clients – known as Intended Parents – contact her every day. She represented the couple in the case of the twins born in India, a case that made legal history. Many of her clients are gay men but not all. Most of them are people who have tried to adopt and have given up.

We begin by asking if we can do surrogacy in the UK. Natalie confirms what my internet searches have already revealed: surrogacy isn't illegal in the UK but commercial surrogacy is illegal and so surrogates can only be paid 'reasonable expenses'. In addition, it's difficult to find a surrogate in the UK because it's illegal to advertise. And the process is risky because surrogacy contracts are not enforceable. If a dispute arises, then the courts are likely to find in favour of the surrogate mother, not the Intended Parents.

In the US the system is different. You can advertise for a surrogate and surrogates can be paid. If there is a dispute, the law will find in favour of the Intended Parents. But can a couple from the UK bring a US surrogate baby back to the UK legally? And will the baby belong to them in law? Natalie starts to explain and the answer sounds like a thorn hedge twenty feet high, dense and prickly. The kind of thorn hedge that exists in fairy tales: when you cut one branch down another grows.

I'm soon lost in the details but Stephen isn't. He makes notes, asks questions, nails the essential difficulties. After all, this is his job. And, as a lawyer, he will risk his whole career if he becomes involved in anything illegal. When finally the conversation ends, it seems that we can – probably, hopefully, maybe – bring a US surrogate baby into the UK without breaking the law. But before we can stick to the law, we will have to make it. This is a world without a map.

Natalie makes it clear that it'll be expensive and that we'll finish up in the High Court. We'll need to write a twenty-page statement so that we can get a Parental Order making the baby legally ours. Stephen brushes aside all these difficulties. He has spent the last four years being misinformed and confused by the medical profession. Now, at last, he's in a world he understands. If there is a legal route then, with Natalie, he's going to find it.

As we drive home, I agree that we can push ahead with this plan, at least for the moment. I'm not worried because I know that some insurmountable obstacle will soon arise. I find it interesting to understand more about surrogacy but I know we'll never go ahead. All we are doing is getting through a few more days.

Winter turns up again. The UK is hit by serious flooding. An inquiry is ordered into our country's involvement in the Iraq War. I put the washing machine on, hang clothes on the line, load the dishwasher, go to the first night of one of my plays, head over to Oxford to teach, curl up with Thomas on the sofa on rainy Sunday afternoons and watch bad DVDs.

We make contact with an American surrogacy agency in Minnesota called the International Assisted Reproduction Center. The young woman who runs the agency is called Keely Snyder and she works with her father, Steve, who is a surrogacy lawyer and a member of the American Bar Association. Stephen feels confident about IARC because of Steve's reputation. Our communication with Keely is by e-mail and occasional conference calls. I'm not familiar with conference calls but Stephen is and so the surrogacy question comes to seem corporate, business-like, part of his work.

We make these calls from Stephen's study during the evening due to the time difference, and our need to hide from Thomas's ever flapping ears. The issues that we discuss with IARC are ridiculously personal and morally complex. They ask – When the birth is taking place, will you want to be fully involved, or would you be happy to remain positioned near the surrogate's head? What if the baby turns out to have severe abnormalities and you want to end the pregnancy and the surrogate doesn't? What if the surrogate is having sex with her husband at the time that the embryos are implanted and she gets pregnant with his baby instead of yours?

I ask the obvious question – What happens if a surrogate mother decides to keep the baby? Keely tells us that IARC have been involved in hundreds of surrogacy arrangements and they've never seen this happen. They select and screen surrogates carefully. The surrogate knows from the beginning that she has no legal claim to the baby. As a gestational surrogate, she also has no genetic link. All the details both legal and emotional are negotiated thoroughly at the beginning. There won't be a problem.

After we put the phone down, Stephen and I stare at each other, raise the palms of our hands, pull faces as though the study ceiling is about to fall down, half-laugh. But I have to hand it to Keely and her colleagues – there is no subject that they can't discuss with frankness and tact.

At the end of these calls the IARC staff say – Have a good day.

After the phone is put down I say – What if this is a hoax? But Stephen transfers money so that IARC can begin the process of finding us a surrogate. Will we ever hear from them again? Or will they just withdraw the funds from the bank and have a good day with our money? I remain convinced that none of this can possibly work because surely there are no women who want to have babies for other women?

I realise that I should be doing more research, talking to a range of different agencies, comparing the costs, understanding the legal situations in different states – because surrogacy law is different in each state. Most people go to California for surrogacy and I should find out why. But I just keep talking to IARC because they keep saying yes. And that's what I need. This whole plan is like one of the fantastic and fragile paper castles, with their mass of tapering spires, which Thomas likes to make out of the inside of loo rolls and tissue paper. If someone blows on it – ever so softly – then the paper will topple and the whole structure will come tumbling down. No more pizza for the penguins.

Reality must not be allowed to arrive. And so I don't say anything to anyone. I know that people will think that what we're doing is weird, extreme, desperate, sad. And I just can't bear to hear it. Please, please just let me continue to build my paper castle. But like every other deceiver, I can't stop myself flirting with the truth. And so, one morning, having coffee with a group of women, I introduce the issue of egg donation without admitting that I have a personal interest in it. One woman says – Oh my God, how could you ever explain that to a child? I mean, that child would just finish up so messed up.

But still I can't stop myself mentioning the question of surrogacy. The response is even less enthusiastic. My fellow coffee drinkers say – I just don't understand it. I mean, what kind of woman could have a baby and hand it over to someone else?

I go home, curl up in bed, cry. Next weekend I go to visit my mum at the farm and ask her what she thinks. Mum is in her seventies now and she's never been to America. She's never used a computer or a mobile phone. In her day IVF didn't exist and infertility was not an issue that could ever be discussed. So it's complicated to explain to her what we're planning to do. But she listens carefully and takes it all in and then she looks at me very directly with her bright blue eyes, and says – You should do it. If you can do, you should. Of course.

Then I go and see Anna in Amberley, the friend who was so kind when I met her in the school corridor. She is now pregnant with her third child but nothing is straightforward. The pregnancy is high risk. She travels to London every week to see a specialist, lives from one day to the next, but still she has time for my questions.

Yes, she says. You should do it. You need to. It will work.

Will it?

Well, it works for all of those celebrities, doesn't it?

As I have no post-Brontë cultural references, I'm unaware of what celebrities do, but Anna fills me in on the details.

It will be horribly expensive, I say.

Yes – but you have the money. And what else are you going to spend it on? Do it. No question. You've got to.

IARC arrange for us to speak to a Norwegian couple on the phone who have surrogate twins. The guy is called Hans and he sounds like someone Stephen might meet through work, or like a dad on the school run. He tells us all about the experience and says that it worked fine for them. At the end of the call we thank him and he says – We don't mind at all. We often talk to people about this. You'll find that if you do surrogacy you finish up becoming an Ambassador for it.

After Stephen and I have put the phone down I say – Would we ever become Ambassadors for surrogacy?

No, he says. But I think we might want to provide a corrective to some of the misinformation around the place.

IARC ask us to prepare a statement explaining our history and identifying the qualities we would look for in a gestational surrogate. I have no idea how to do this but I type something up and also e-mail the requested photographs. Almost immediately IARC send back a short document giving details of a potential gestational surrogate.

Her name is Amanda and she has a partner who is also called Amanda, or Manda. They have a six-year-old daughter and live in a small town in Minnesota. A fuzzy photograph of Amanda shows her wearing jeans and a fleece and looking – normal. Stephen and I don't need to discuss whether the fact that Amanda is in a single-sex relationship is a problem because we both know that it isn't.

Stephen and I look through the document again together. Apparently Amanda wants to be a gestational surrogate because she likes having babies and she and Manda want some money so that they can have treatment to have their own baby. We ask IARC if this is normal. If Amanda wants a baby herself then why wouldn't she just keep our baby? IARC assure us that women often donate eggs or become surrogates in order to fund fertility treatment. This doesn't seem right. Does the State not fund treatment for Amanda and Manda? No. Because this is America, where people stitch up their own wounds because they have no medical insurance.

Stephen and I are both thinking the same – have Amanda and Manda not heard of the turkey baster? Can't they just find a man who is willing to donate some sperm and then shoot it up? That's what gay women usually do, isn't it? Maybe they don't have turkey basters in America?

IARC organise for us to speak to Amanda on the telephone. I imagine that she will be loud and talkative because all

Americans are, aren't they? But Amanda is quietly spoken and sounds shy. Immediately we have the feeling that we like her. She talks about her daughter Olivia, her partner Manda and their interest in pit bull terriers.

Pit bulls have a bad reputation, Amanda says, but they really don't deserve it. Usually they just haven't been treated properly. Amanda works as a volunteer for a charity which takes in abandoned pit bulls, rehabilitates them and finds new homes. Stephen and I can do Dog Conversations and Animal Rescue Conversations because of my mother. And so the phone call runs on smoothly enough.

Amanda is a churchgoer and her surrogacy plan has the support of her congregation. She admits that she doesn't eat a good diet and is trying to improve. She suggests that, once she's pregnant, we should send a CD of some music that we like. She can play that around the house and then the baby will hopefully feel at home when he or she goes to England. This is all moving too fast for me.

Amanda talks about how she will explain the surrogacy to her daughter, Olivia. It's the same as the pit bulls, she says. We have a pit bull we own and then there are others who are boarders. This baby will be a boarder as well, coming to stay until he or she goes to a new home.

Fine, no problem.

I don't know how you can decide that you like someone when you've only spoken to them on the phone for twenty minutes, but we do decide. Are we just desperate? Or simply overwhelmed by the idea of what this unknown woman is offering to do for us? I don't know but I trust Amanda. As for the pit bulls, I find it a little strange to find my future baby compared to a delinquent dog, but if the logic works for Amanda, then it works for me.

The next stage is to find an egg donor. Simple. I'll get in touch with the cello-playing German woman with the long fingers. But, of course, it doesn't work like that. Instead IARC give us the details of their own database that contains information on approximately one hundred and fifty young women who work for them as egg donors. All, we are assured, have been carefully screened.

These women are white, black, Asian, divorced, single, married, short, tall, fat, thin. Some are mothers, some aren't. Some have donated eggs before, some haven't. The database gives a photograph of each woman and options to click for further information. No names are given but each woman has a reference that begins with OV and is followed by a three figure number.

These references bother me, the whole database bothers me. I've never been on a dating website but maybe they look like this? Perhaps there's always something humiliating about people selling themselves, no matter what part of themselves they're selling? Some of the women seem to have mistaken the egg donation process for a glamour modelling audition. Professionally taken photographs show them in cut-off T-shirts with smooth midriffs, blonde hair piled on their heads and too much make-up.

But perhaps their confusion is understandable. After all, how do you advertise yourself as having desirable genes? Other photographs are blurred or show women with hats pulled down over their eyes. Some women have included photographs of their children. Their professions are home-maker, beautician, business administrator, nurse or fitness instructor.

The database also gives endless information about the women's health and the health of others in their family. A great-aunt died of cancer, a maternal grandmother was short-sighted, an aunt died young in an accident, a second cousin has asthma. The database reveals nothing and everything. Stephen and I agree that we aren't interested in the medical details. Any baby which is alive will do fine for us.

Do you actually know whether your maternal grandmother was short-sighted? I ask.

No, Stephen says. I admit to being similarly uncertain.

I continue to look through the database even though it makes my skin shrink. Had we adopted a baby, then I would have been happy to have a baby girl of any size, colour, shape or race. If we had used a donor egg in England or in Spain then we would have had no choice – and no possibility of finding out anything about the donor. So now it seems wrong to choose. *Daily Mail* headlines ring through my mind. *Designer Babies for Sale. Couple order six foot blonde with PhD.*

I consider ringing IARC and asking them to stick a pin in the list for us. But then I think again. Since we're being offered the choice then why not take it? I think of friends in Brussels who have adopted children of other races. Those adoptions have all worked well, but I sometimes think that it must be complicated for those couples and their children, dealing with the enquiring glances in the street, having to explain it all again and again. So if Stephen and I have the opportunity to have a child who looks like us then, for the sake of the child, shouldn't we take it?

I look through the database again, but I'm tired and the choice confuses me. Why are we doing this anyway? This whole surrogacy idea was never meant to be serious. If only one of the five had stayed alive. If only we didn't have to do all this.

Finally I say to Stephen – Look, what do you want? Brains or beauty?

No one should ever have to ask a question like this.

Brains, Stephen says, without hesitating. And someone who looks like you.

So I search for pale, slim, well educated, medium height. That doesn't work. Few of the women are particularly well educated. By definition, highly educated women probably don't sell their eggs. So I simplify the search: pale and approximately five foot six. This brings up ten women and I look at them in more detail. None of the photographs appeals to me. Yesterday I felt I was being offered too much choice, now I feel as though I'm being offered too little. Is there another database? *Everything's free in America, for a small fee in America.* I mourn for the German woman with the long fingers and the promising music career.

The agency realise that we are having difficulty deciding and suggest that we check the database on Friday afternoons because that's when new details are posted up. As I follow their advice, I'm reminded of when I was young and looking for a flat in London, how I rushed to buy the *Evening Standard* as soon as it came out, scurried through the property pages, then furiously fed ten pence pieces into the call box.

But Fridays come and go and still we fail to make a decision. Perhaps it doesn't matter anyway? I just want a baby, I don't care what the baby looks likes. Stephen is telling me that we just need to pick someone, anyone. Friday comes again but I'm losing hope and don't bother to check the database until Saturday morning. At first I think that there are no new details – but then I see her and I know her immediately. The woman I want.

There's nothing exceptional about her but her girl-next-door face is illuminated by a humorous, intelligent smile.

She wears a baseball cap and carries a rucksack. She looks carefree, energetic, a citizen of the world, even though she is probably only walking to the end of the block. In another photograph, she's turned sideways and a cascade of luscious hair falls down over her shoulder. That appeals to me because, in my family, we may not be beautiful but we have good hair.

I read more about this baseball-capped woman – she's of Estonian origin and she's a nurse with a Bachelor's degree in science. She's married with triplets and she doesn't want more children. She likes reading and crafts, as I do. The photograph of her triplets shows three laughing tots sitting in a bubble-filled bath. So that's it: world traveller, a good head of hair, a reader with happy, normal kids. But when I contact IARC, some other Intended Parents have already paid the deposit and moved their furniture in.

I go to bed in tears. Why are we even considering this? The whole plan is ridiculous. We don't know even one other person who has done this, anywhere. I just want my life back, I want to write my book and move on. I need to focus on Thomas. He is more than enough for me. But then, three days later, IARC call and say that the other Intended Parents have pulled out and the egg donor with the baseball cap is willing to work with us.

Still one problem remains. Does this egg donor want to remain anonymous or is there a chance that she is prepared to have a little direct contact with us? IARC are happy to ask this question, but they warn that this will involve further costs, further legal agreements. We instruct them to ask the question and to send the egg donor the profile that we prepared for Amanda.

In particular, I want this egg donor to know that we are far away in England. She will never meet us in the street, we will never drop in on her. I also ask IARC to explain that we don't expect much contact: a name, an address, occasional photographs, a Christmas card. And also the possibility for our child to meet her some day if the need arises. To me, all this is important because when that child asks about his or her genetic mother I want to be able to give a reasonable level of information. I wait in fear for a response.

Good news. Yes, this egg donor is happy to have some level of contact with us. All we have to do is wait for the relevant legal agreements to be put in place then we can get in touch with her directly. I'm amazed by the courage of this woman whose name I don't know. She might one day have to tell her three children that she is an egg donor and that there is a child who is genetically related to them living in England. And she runs the risk that many years into the future she will open her front door and find a young man or woman on her doorstep who is – at least genetically – her child. I'm overwhelmed with gratitude that she's prepared to do this for us.

IARC ring to say that Steve Snyder will be in London and suggest that we should meet him. The timing is not convenient. Thomas is playing in a concert at school that afternoon. Stephen and I hastily agree that I will go to the concert and he will go to the meeting. Steve Snyder is in London for an event called the Fertility Fair.

Fair? I say. Fair? You mean, like goldfish in plastic bags, candy floss, and a waltzer?

Yes, Stephen says. Probably. But maybe not goldfish. More like a coconut shy and if you knock all the coconuts down then you win a baby.

But, as so often happens in the modern world, satire is

rendered irrelevant because no matter how much you might exaggerate a situation, reality will turn out to be more extreme. Stephen returns from his trip to the Fertility Fair.

No coconut shy, he says. But there was a raffle. And the prize was a free cycle of IVF.

I start laughing wildly and then stop.

I don't actually find any of this funny, I say.

Stephen puts his arms around me. I know, he says.

I shrug and we agree that it is difficult being stiff, pale English people adrift in the surreal world of American infertility. Meanwhile the paperwork keeps coming and we keep signing it. Our signatures always need to be witnessed and so often I drive across the Common, late at night, or early in the morning, to Anna's house in Amberley. As she is a lawyer, she can act as a witness. When I arrive she is usually breastfeeding her new baby, pouring milk onto Weetabix for the boys, hanging out the washing. But still she always signs everything that needs signing. If we were in our right minds, we would not be doing any of this.

I drive to Hay-on-Wye to see Joslin. I set off early and it's a fine morning. When I arrive Hay is decked out in sunshine and new summer green. Joslin has no hair and she's wearing a back brace and yet strangely she is beautiful. Ellie is sitting at a table playing with Joslin's pills. There are hundreds of them in a rainbow of colours and they come in a special box with endless tiny compartments.

I know I shouldn't let her play with them, Joslin says. But they're exactly what a little girl wants to play with, aren't they? Such deadly beauty.

We sit in the tiny back garden, in the sun. Joslin tells me about her morning. Ellie and James are looking after a hamster for the weekend that belongs to the school. All the children in the class get their chance to care for the hamster. Understandably, Joslin didn't really want the hamster but, of course, she couldn't say no.

So seven o'clock this morning I hear the kids making all this noise downstairs, she says. And I really don't want to get up but there's no choice. So I come downstairs and Ellie has decided that the hamster cage needs cleaning out. What can I say to her? She's trying to do the right thing, except the only problem is that we have no new bedding. And Ellie has already efficiently emptied all the old bedding into the bin. Disaster. What can I do? I've got no choice. I have to find an old newspaper and empty the contents of the bin onto the floor. And then I have to sort through the rubbish and the hamster poo in order to find the clean bits of the bedding. And I have to pick them out and put them back in the cage.

Joslin is convulsed by laughter but also winces in pain.

So there I am, she says. It's seven o'clock in the morning and I haven't even had a coffee. And I have terminal cancer – and that's what I'm doing.

I love Joslin so much.

Later she says – This week, after the chemotherapy, I felt so bad that I didn't care if I lost my life. And I realised that's probably how people die, how I'll die. You reach a level of pain where you just won't want to live any more. I've been wondering exactly how it happens – and I think that's the way it goes.

XXI

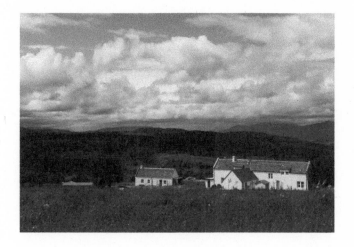

The test of a first rate intelligence is the ability to hold two opposed ideas in the mind at the same time and still retain the ability to function.

F. Scott Fitzgerald – 'The Crack-up'

What exactly is the problem with surrogacy? Finally I think it comes down to the fact that many people – most people perhaps – don't believe that a woman should be able to give birth to a baby and then hand that baby over to another woman. If you can do that then surely you aren't a proper woman? But who defines what a proper woman is?

Answer – men do. Or at least they have done for the last two millennia. That may be changing but you can't shift ideas developed over thousands of years in the space of two generations. And so our idea about women is essentially still male and Christian. The Virgin Mary. The happy, selfless mother. A woman untainted by the stain of personal gain, of money.

But do I know any women like this? My friends on the school run have dishwater hands and broken nails. Tough and vital, they can wipe the bottom of their senile mother with one hand while cooking dinner for eight with the other. They may need protection but they don't get it. Instead they protect men from all the grisly bits. Life, death, blocked drains.

For these women, real women, life is mucky and full of unacceptable compromises. It involves doing things a proper woman shouldn't do. So is surrogacy wrong, or are the images that supposedly characterise women wildly inaccurate? Once again, it comes down to the yawning gap between our lives as reflected by the media and our lives as actually lived.

But this isn't the only problem with surrogacy. There is another problem, thornier and knottier, a problem that has to do with money and class, issues which English people don't like to discuss. The truth is that, in general, surrogacy is something that poor women do for rich women. Rich women do not become surrogate mums. And surrogacy is usually too expensive even for people with average incomes.

Stephen and I have navigated our way around this question by going to America, where we hope that people are less likely to do things just for money. Overall this assumption is probably not correct – but at least in America we can find individuals who we know are not making decisions dictated entirely by financial need. But then the very reason why we're going to America is because we have the money to avoid the moral complexity of India or the Ukraine.

The world is full of inequalities. Poor women clean the houses of rich women. Poor women look after the children of affluent women, sometimes neglecting their own children in the process. Is surrogacy different? Do the income inequalities make it morally wrong? The English legal system gets around this question by banning commercial surrogacy. But this simply means that people go abroad. Or it leads to a situation where a woman does the most important job ever for another woman – for free. Is this an act of selfless love offered by a pure woman? Or is it slave labour? If I refuse to pay my cleaning lady, that makes the inequalities between us worse, not better. If surrogacy is going to exist then shouldn't it at least be fairly remunerated? It is perfectly possible to love and be paid for it.

And on top of all that, the whole surrogacy business smells of some futuristic, science-fiction world in which an elite of women occupy themselves with higher tasks while an underclass of women do the dirty stuff, like bringing babies into the world. A world in which some women are not only Too Posh To Push, as the tabloids like to say, but are so posh that they spurn the basic business of pregnancy itself and hand it over to someone else.

But now the morality of surrogacy is the least of our worries because the whole plan has gone wrong, as I always knew it would. I'm away from home for a week, teaching for the Arvon Foundation at Moniack Mhor, north of Inverness. Some weeks ago, a date was fixed for Stephen and me to talk to a doctor in Canada. He's a doctor with whom IARC have worked many times before and they're sure that he will be the right person to help us.

When these arrangements were made it didn't even occur to Stephen and me to point out that the date would be inconvenient. For months now we've taken calls at any time of the day or night. Because I know that it's unlikely that my mobile will work at Moniack Mhor, I've arranged with Arvon to take a break from work and use their office phone when the call comes.

And so here I am, on a Wednesday afternoon, in a white-walled croft in Scotland, sitting in the tiny office that adjoins the main buildings of the centre. From the window of the office, I can see sheep grazing behind a wire fence and behind them miles of Scottish moorland, purple and grey in the August drizzle. I've been waiting a long time for the call now, reading a book to steady my nerves.

Finally Stephen rings me to check that I'm ready for the call. Then IARC ring us to say that there is a delay. Again I read my book, waiting, hearing the distant voices of my students chatting in the kitchen. Finally the call from Canada comes in. The doctor we are speaking to asks – How is the weather where you are?

Stephen explains that he's in Gloucestershire and I'm in Scotland. Cordial jokes are cracked about how this conception plan is now spanning three countries. I join in the pleasantries although in some bitter part of my mind I'm thinking – I would have been more than happy with a conception that took place after a drunken evening in the pub, or in a holiday hotel. I never wanted a child conceived on a three-way conference call.

The doctor begins by asking us about the medical information which we have submitted. To begin with everything seems to go smoothly but then we move onto legal issues. Stephen is asking more and more questions and he isn't getting the answers he wants. I think of that thorn hedge in fairy tales – every time you cut away a branch, it grows again. The call grinds to a halt. My mind has become scrambled. I don't even understand exactly what the problem is but I do understand that we can't proceed. I'm bent double over the desk in front of me, like someone who's been punched in the stomach. Stephen thanks the doctor and tells me to put the phone down.

Immediately he rings back. I'm wailing quietly. We can neither of us understand what's happened. We can't cut through the forest of thorns. The paper castle has collapsed. Stephen tries to calm me down and says that he will talk to IARC and get back to me. I return to my teaching, try to make it appear as though nothing has happened. But I'm numb and shocked. Why have we been told that this is possible when it isn't? We should have gone to an agency in California instead.

It isn't until late that night that Stephen manages to reach me on his mobile. He's spoken to IARC and they're as surprised as we are. It had never occurred to them that there might be a problem. Slowly Stephen and I are realising that, although IARC represent themselves as having plenty of experience of international surrogacy, in fact, we're their first English clients.

There is no system, no instruction manual, no map. We always knew this but it's a shock to find that our American friends are as lost as we are. But IARC aren't going to give up and neither is Stephen. So he's agreed with them that they'll try and find another clinic. Stephen and I are also worried that Amanda will desert us. After all, she wants to go ahead with a surrogate pregnancy. It would be far easier for her to find some Intended Parents in America.

Speaking to Stephen should make me feel better. After all, it is still possible that we can go to another clinic – but I can't stop crying. I've never believed in the surrogacy plan but, now that it's slipping away from us, I realise that a part of me had put faith in it. I lie awake in the narrow Arvon single bed and stare out at the night sky – wide and infinitely black – and listen to the silence of the Scottish moorland all around.

Now that the plan has started unravelling, it unspools endlessly. IARC try again and again to find us another clinic. Throughout the autumn of 2010, our paperwork travels across the States from one clinic to another. First it's New Jersey but, under the law of that state, Stephen's sperm would be considered to be an animal import and would therefore be subject to the laws covering BSE. As a result, his sperm would need to be quarantined for six months and would therefore be unusable.

After that: Los Angeles. I imagine our baby in a show girl's tutu, dancing in a chorus line. But Los Angeles can't help either. And so it goes on. One clinic after another. I think of those American road movies – huge cars, long, straight roads, cutting through endless miles of dust, the horizons bounded by red rocks. Our imagined baby travelling around the States, trying to find a place where she can legally be born. A cheerleader, a cow girl, a beach bumming Californian babe.

And all the time I'm waiting to hear that Amanda has

grown tired of waiting, that our egg donor has decided to sign up with another couple. But Keely at IARC says again and again – Don't worry. Amanda is fine. Your donor is fine. They're both going to wait for as long as it takes.

I receive news that Joslin has been taken into a hospice. I panic, assuming this means that she's dying, but soon discover that hospices are not only for the dying, they also care for people who are seriously ill and need some time away from their families. The hospice is at Bartestree, on the road between Ledbury and Hereford, only fifteen miles from my mum's farm, a shorter drive for me than either Hay-on-Wye or Hereford.

The hospice is modern and hushed, as pleasant as such a place can be. The carpets are muted turquoise, flecked with purple and the doors and handrails are all pale wood. The walls are hung with tasteful watercolours of flowers and slumbering landscapes. I smile at everybody and everybody beams back. As I walk the corridors towards Joslin's room, an elderly lady with a Zimmer frame sits with her friend near a door that leads out into the garden.

I might be dying, the lady says. But I'm not sure. I hope I am. Perhaps I should stand up.

Joslin's room looks out over a concrete terrace, a functional iron balcony. A white rose twists and climbs through the metalwork, its flowers nodding and shedding leaves onto the concrete. Beyond the balcony is a sloping field newly planted with apple trees. They stand in straight rows on bright green grass.

You know, Joslin says, I used to find that every bit of happiness I had was undercut by the knowledge that I am dying. So I used to look out at the garden and see the children playing and I would think – isn't it beautiful to see that? But then I would think – but I am dying. But now it's different, better. Because I've learnt that you need to change the word But for the word And. So now I say – It's beautiful to see the children playing in the garden *and* I'm dying. It's such a small change but so significant.

Later we manage to get out into the garden. Joslin can walk about fifty yards on sticks although it hurts her to do so. We sit down on a bench shaded by a creeper and trees. A woman comes towards us on sticks. She has carefully tended grey hair, a sparkling smile, but her eyes are hungry as a hunter. She has us in her sights and is determined to speak. I feel torn. Doubtless this woman is dying and so we should take the time and trouble to chat to her, to listen to her story. I promised Laura, I have to look after the suffering.

But Joslin is surprisingly firm. Lovely to see you. But not right now, Edith, because I'm talking to my friend. I'll drop in on you later.

Edith offers surprisingly little resistance, backs off and shuffles away.

I tell Joslin that I admire her ability to put someone off like that.

Oh God, she says. You've got to. In a place like this everyone is a bad news story. You'd lose your mind if you didn't know how to get rid of them – pleasantly.

She's silent for a minute and then says – But you need them as well.

And she tells me then how lonely she is. She does sometimes go to the hospice support group. She met a woman she liked there called Jean. Jean was in her fifties, intelligent and funny, a former theatre director. She had decided to blow all her savings on a Morgan sports car, something she had always dreamed of having.

Then she'd set off on trips around England, the Highlands of Scotland, the Welsh coast. Just driving and driving, enjoying the roar of the car and the endlessly changing scenery. She'd sent Joslin texts with pictures of herself standing by the car in front of castles, cliffs, hotels, sunsets. And she'd come back to the hospice a couple of times, thin and luminous, gripping more photos. But then Jean didn't show up again and Joslin doesn't know what happened, although it isn't hard to guess.

That's the thing, Joslin says. It can be difficult to make lasting friendships in a hospice support group. I liked Jean, the car. Imagine driving and driving, coming to a junction, and thinking – right, left? And you could go anywhere. Anywhere at all.

Burmese opposition politician Aung San Suu Kyi is finally released. WikiLeaks spills American diplomatic secrets all across the internet. The days come at me like the headlights of oncoming cars, dazzling bright for a moment and then gone. I put the washing machine on, hang clothes on the line, walk with Thomas along the seafront at Weston-super-Mare, write.

Finally IARC tell us that they have solved our problem. Dr Yatsenko in San Diego, California, now has all our paperwork and he's prepared to help us. He's worked with English couples before, and he sees no reason why he can't work with us. He has read all the information about both Amanda and our donor and is satisfied that they are both suitable for the roles they intend to perform.

We speak to Dr Yatsenko on the phone and he explains to us how everything will work. Firstly the egg donor's menstrual cycle will be aligned with Amanda's menstrual cycle. Then Stephen will need to go to California to make a sperm donation. After that, eggs will be harvested from the donor, fertilised with Stephen's sperm and then implanted in Amanda. The way that Dr Yatsenko explains it makes it all sound simple and normal. And so a date is set for Stephen to go to California in January 2011. But still I know that this will never happen.

Christmas comes and surrogacy is all over the British newspapers because Elton John and his partner have travelled with their son, born to a US surrogate mum, back to the UK. Opinions are bandied around. *Why didn't they adopt? It should be made illegal. No, it shouldn't. It's their business, they can do what they like. OK. OK. But shouldn't a child have both a father and a mother?*

I don't read much of the press coverage and I don't say anything to anyone. My mum knows, Anna in Amberley and Joslin know, but no one else has any idea at all – and I can't think how I would begin to explain it to them.

XXII

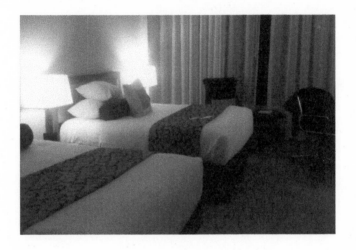

Love and work. Work and love.
That's all there is.

Freud

It's the middle of January 2011 and Stephen is leaving for San Diego to meet Dr Yatsenko in just a few days. I realise that I have no idea what we're doing. I may have engaged in the legal and administrative aspects of surrogacy, but I know nothing about how a surrogate pregnancy works. Elton John presumably knows, but I don't feel able to call up and ask.

In particular, I'm worried that I haven't been in touch with Amanda enough. What if she doubts our commitment or support? But what do I say to her? I sign up for internet message boards and read furiously. And what is it that I find? Certainly no trailer parks or reality TV shows. No Intended Parents fighting through the courts to get the surrogate mum to hand over the baby.

Instead a world of women who are sincerely trying to help other women with this problem which only a woman can fully understand. A warm and supportive world, a world full of good news stories. But also a secret world, embattled, defensive. All of these women protect their identities carefully because they're frightened of being misunderstood. So why do they do what they do?

Leanne from Texas: I became a surrogate because I just love, love, love having babies. So after my husband and I had our two, I just felt gutted because we really, really didn't want more children and yet I just couldn't bear not to do it again – and so it was logical for me to do it for another woman. I've been a gestational surrogate three times now and I think I'll do it one more time at least. People think it's weird and they think it's just about money – but it's none of their business.

Siobhan from California: I decided to become a surrogate mum after watching my sister and her husband do IVF ten times. Their marriage was a wreck and it was really hard for everyone in our family. When they finally managed to adopt, it was such a huge miracle for everyone and such a relief. Now I just want to help another family avoid all that pain.

Jenny writes: I'm a surrogate because I really want to stay home with my three young children but I can't afford it. Through surrogacy I'm helping another family and I'm also managing to give my children a great childhood. And I like being pregnant. I know from the beginning that the baby I'm carrying isn't mine, so although I love that baby, I never really feel any attachment and have felt no problem in saying goodbye.

Kiley writes: I feel so blessed by Jesus. I have two lovely children, a great husband, a comfortable home. I want to put something back, but with a family to raise I can't do the Peace Corps. Surrogacy is my way of saying thank you. People in my family don't understand but I don't care. My husband supports me and that's all that matters. Once I gave an interview to a journalist. I'll never do that again because he made me sound like an uneducated slut trying to make a quick buck.

And the Intended Parents – who are they? Most of them are couples who have battled long and hard with infertility. Many of them have health problems that make it hard for them to carry a child. A significant number suffer from MKRH Syndrome, a condition which means that they have ovaries and produce eggs but they have no uterus and so can never carry a baby.

One woman from Connecticut writes that she was diagnosed with MKRH aged thirteen when her periods didn't start. Everyone in her family was so upset that they decided, there and then, to raise the money so that she would be able to do surrogacy when she was older. Once people in the neighbourhood heard about the MKRH they all raised money as well. So when she got married the money was there for her to have two children using a surrogate mum.

She now has those two children, a boy and a girl, aged five and three. Genetically they are her children and her husband's. But she feels as though her children belong to her whole community because so many people raised money to help bring them into the world.

Then there are the stories of how the surrogacy actually happens. Most of them are about the American surrogacy system and begin with an agency, a lawyer, a clinic. But in countries where the surrogacy laws are more restrictive, it soon becomes clear that some strange things go on. The most extraordinary story comes from Doreen in Kent.

Doreen and her husband Sam tried IVF five times. Then they tried to adopt from China but, after waiting four years, they started to give up hope. And so Doreen posted a message on the internet offering £20,000 for a surrogate. In doing this, Doreen knew that she was breaking the law twice over – firstly by advertising for a surrogate and secondly by offering to pay. But Doreen had reached the stage when she didn't care.

She didn't expect a reply to her advert but soon a woman called Karen in Scotland got in touch. Karen had three children but her marriage had recently broken up and she needed to make some money. She'd always liked the idea of surrogacy – so why not? This was to be traditional surrogacy and Karen was happy with that. And so Doreen and Sam remortgaged their house and an arrangement was made. Everyone involved was sworn to secrecy.

Having already borrowed heavily, Doreen and Sam had no money to waste and Karen agreed that they should try to keep things as cheap as possible. And so it was agreed that, when Karen ovulated, they would all meet up in Doncaster. The plan was to book a hotel room where Sam would provide the sperm and Karen the turkey baster. Then perhaps lunch afterwards.

But when the day came there was heavy snow and the trains from Scotland were delayed. Karen wasn't sure whether she should set off, but Sam and Doreen pleaded with her to give it a try. Sam had only been able to get one day off work and so he and Doreen couldn't delay. They reached Doncaster without any trouble, but the texts they received from Karen on her southbound train weren't encouraging. The snow was still coming down and trains were being cancelled. But still Karen was hoping she might reach them in time.

Sam and Doreen waited and waited in the freezing cold, pacing up and down the platform at Doncaster Station. Their return train to Kent would leave at 17.30 and, if they missed it, they would have to pay for another ticket. Karen sent a text from Newcastle at 11.30 and another from Leeds at 14.30. Her train was now due in at Doncaster at 16.00. But finally that train didn't arrive until 16.45. It was clear that no hotel room would be possible. Instead matters had to be dealt with in the station toilets, with Doreen waiting outside the doors of the men's loos to carry the tube of sperm into Karen in the ladies' loos.

Amazingly Karen did fall pregnant as a result of this strange transaction and everything then went ahead as planned. Baby David was born safely with Doreen and Sam travelling to Scotland for the birth. Due to the hospital regulations, he had to be handed over in the car park outside the hospital, which was less than ideal, and Doreen had to engage in a lot of deceit to explain to the authorities in her area how she came to have a baby. But Doreen, Sam and Karen are all pleased by the outcome and still very much in touch. Karen is hoping to do the same thing again for another couple – although she'll make more flexible travel arrangements another time.

Although Doreen has posted her story on the internet, understandably she doesn't tell it to many people in her real life. Her name isn't really Doreen, her husband isn't Sam. But one day she will tell the story to David – or most of it anyway. Perhaps not the bit about Doncaster Station. Because, after all, conception is meant to be a private business. As Doreen says, we all want to believe that we were conceived in love. That we were absolutely wanted, intended. Doncaster Station doesn't have the right ambience.

But then the truth is that many of us were probably conceived thoughtlessly after a drunken night at the pub, or as a result of sex that was less than satisfactory. Maybe Doncaster Station is not so bad? I don't know. What I do know is that conception is best kept secret, but that, unfortunately, assisted reproduction lays it bare. Even a Saturday night knee-trembler in an alleyway does involve passion – however brief.

Doreen's story fascinates me – but it's a distraction I can't afford. All this reading is helpful, but still I haven't managed to find one couple in England who has experience of surrogacy in the US. Finally I pluck up courage, master the technology and type a message onto an American website under the heading 'International'. A few days later I check the website and am amazed to find a message.

It's from a woman in North Yorkshire called Charlotte who has surrogate twins who are two and a half years old. She gives me her phone number, tells me it's fine to call that evening. We are snowed in, yet again. When I speak to Charlotte she is snowed in as well and her day has been complicated. A man's car has skidded on the ice and crashed through their garden wall. But still she's got time to talk.

I feel as though I've reached an oasis in the desert. Charlotte immediately feels like an old friend. She and her husband did surrogacy because she had breast cancer and was told that she would never be able to have children. At the time no legal framework existed at all, so she simply organised everything in America and brought the babies home through Heathrow with no questions asked. I'm thrilled to find out that she also went to Dr Yatsenko and is full of praise for him.

He just can't get it, she laughs. He can't see what we find odd about it.

Charlotte is still in touch with their surrogate mum and met briefly with their egg donor, although she found that difficult.

Was it weird? I ask. Going to America to fetch your sons.

Yes, she says. Very. The girls came early and we missed the birth. And so we left in a rush and arrived in the rain in the middle of the night in this American city and parked in the car park of this hospital. And yes, it was strange. But then we went into the hospital and we saw the girls and they were ours and I knew it. And after that it was easy.

As we end our call, she says – You know, at the time it just all seemed so extreme. But now I'm just a normal mother with normal twin girls going to the mother and toddler group and clearing up the Duplo.

I'm looking forward to normal, I say.

Stephen and I have long discussions about whether I should go to San Diego. Initially I feel sure that I should. Although I may be redundant in this process, I don't want to feel redundant. But what would I be going for? We know we're not going to meet either Amanda or our egg donor although they will be visiting the clinic at around the same time. And logistically it will be complicated – who will pick Thomas up from school?

Stephen feels that there's no point in me going. The journey will be endless and expensive and we'll only be there twenty-four hours. Stephen will simply fly to San Diego, go to the clinic and then return. I think back to IVF in Brussels. The nurse who suggested that perhaps I should disappear behind the plastic hospital curtain and give Stephen a hand? Whether it's Brussels or San Diego, the idea is still ridiculous.

I ask if San Diego is near the sea. I'm not missing out on a seaside town even if it does mean sitting on a plane for twelve hours. Stephen tells me that San Diego isn't near the sea. He's wrong, of course, but eventually we agree that I won't go but that he'll send me lots of photos along the way.

And so the morning comes when he's due to leave. I've already dropped Thomas off at school and so we stand together awkwardly in the hall. The moment is both momentous and ordinary. Stephen is always leaving on business trips so why is this one any different? I kiss him goodbye, shrug.

Well, I say. Have a good wank in San Diego.

Stephen sends me grainy mobile phone photographs. Here's the security arch you walk through at the airport, here is the hotel bedroom. The bedside lamps have square shades, the curtains are translucent, a room service menu lies on the bed. The room could be anywhere in the world.

Here is the outside of the clinic. He can't photograph inside the clinic as they don't allow that. I e-mail Amanda to thank her and wish her luck. I also send an e-mail via IARC to our egg donor. Soon we might be in touch with her directly but we're still waiting for the legal process which will allow that to be completed. I try to make the e-mails sound warm and supportive but I'm not sure I've said the right thing. I meet my friend Anna, who has signed so many of the legal papers, for a coffee and she is excited but I can only say – I long to live in uninteresting times.

Three days after Stephen returns from the States, Dr Yatsenko phones to tell us that there are thirteen eggs. Then the next day he phones to say that we have twelve embryos. Stephen and I don't know what this means. Is this what is expected? The clinic seem pleased. Stephen rings with this news as I'm walking down the High Street in Stroud. What happens next? I'm unclear. Is our embryo being taken from the test tube in San Diego and being implanted into Amanda right now?

When I get home, my question is answered. Dr Yatsenko rings to say that the transfer will take place on Sunday. He says that he has two girl embryos and two boys. After that call, Stephen looks worried.

I don't like it, he says. They should say male and female, not boy and girl. I didn't like that when I was there and I told them that.

But we have crossed a line, haven't we? I say.

Yes. But still.

I ask myself – how significant is that line? Eggs have become embryos. Eggs aren't human life. Most women of child-bearing age flush one down the loo each month. But embryos have been fertilised and so could be human lives. Except that one can't see them with the naked eye.

Are they lives? I say.

No, Stephen says. One shouldn't confuse a few cells with human life.

But we're both aware that we now have responsibilities towards these two male embryos. What will happen if we don't use them? We've been told that eventually we could ask for them to be destroyed or we could donate them anonymously. I feel that we should donate them, but once again I find myself worried by the idea of anonymity.

At every turn this becomes more complicated. I read on the internet that there are half a million frozen embryos in the US, half a million lives which could be happening but aren't. This seems a tragedy when those embryos could change the life of a woman battling with infertility. Can we give our embryos to a couple we know? And where would we find such a couple?

Once again I go on the internet. Soon I discover an agency that deals with the adoption of embryos. Is there anything in America for which they don't have an agency? Bizarrely, the Snowflakes Embryo Adoption Agency was set up by Catholics concerned about the growing number of unused embryos. Their role is to match people who may have embryos to give away with couples who need them. I ask Stephen how he feels about giving up embryos for adoption. Unsurprisingly he tells me that it's far too early to talk about any of this.

Dr Yatsenko calls with a question. How many embryos should he implant? I thought we had decided this – only one embryo. But Stephen had conversations in San Diego that have made him reconsider. The statistics go like this – if Amanda is implanted with one egg then she has a 40 per cent chance of getting pregnant. It she is implanted with two eggs then the chances of a pregnancy are over 80 per cent.

But we don't want twins, I say.

Yes, Stephen says. But of that 80 per cent, only 10 per cent will be twins.

It's a difficult one. I still only want one embryo to be implanted but the statistics are persuasive. Stephen feels that maybe we should ask for two embryos because it would be in everyone's best interest if this worked the first time. If it doesn't then he, Amanda and our egg donor will have to go to California again. Finally we agree on two.

On Sunday the call comes as we're walking across Rodborough Common to the ice cream factory. I challenge Thomas to a game of tag so he doesn't hear the call. But then I dodge back towards Stephen and tell him to ask Dr Yatsenko to give Amanda all our love. After that we walk on to the ice cream factory and sit on a bench eating rum and raisin, rhubarb and ginger, mint choc chip. And somewhere in California our child is starting out on the journey towards life.

XXIII

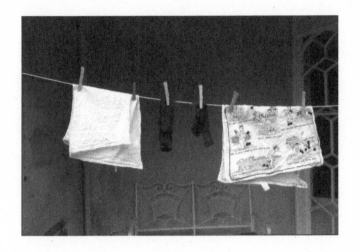

What comes from the heart, goes to the heart.

Samuel Taylor Coleridge

I put the washing machine on, hang clothes on the line, load the dishwasher, throw my novel in the bin and then get it out again. I go to Clevedon and walk on the pier. I help Thomas with his homework and explain to him that no one with black teeth ever gets a girlfriend. So clean your teeth. Now. No, now. Right now.

News comes that on Thursday, 2nd February, Amanda will have the results of the pregnancy test. Due to the time difference, we won't get the news until late at night. Stephen and I put Thomas to bed and get out a boxed set of *Inspector Morse*. We're both Morse fans and have had this boxed set in reserve, ready for an occasion when we need to be thoroughly distracted.

And so we light the fire in the playroom, put on Inspector Morse. And there he is sailing through the streets of Oxford in that maroon car. A don has been murdered and his wife turns out to be an old flame of Morse's. And then Lewis has problems with his wife because he's stayed on late at work and she's missed her Spanish lesson again. And as the soprano wails the aria from *The Magic Flute*, Morse is going to be disappointed in love yet again.

Stephen looks at his mobile and realises that he's missed Dr Yatsenko's call. He listens to the message and tells me that the news is positive and that Dr Yatsenko will ring back. Neither of us react to this information because we don't trust it. I'm still wondering what vital piece of information was in the academic paper that the Oxford don was going to present on the night before he was hit over the head with the marble statuette stolen from the college library.

Stephen has gone to get a glass of wine. The mobile rings again and he dashes back. It slips from his hands, disappears down the back of the sofa. In the process of getting it out, he cuts off the call and when he rings back the number is engaged. I'm close to tears. I suggest putting *Inspector Morse* back on and Stephen tells me to shut up. Finally the phone call comes again.

Amanda is calling us from California. She's there with Manda – and Keely from IARC in Minneapolis is on the call as well. I hadn't known that Amanda was planning to stay on in California. Suddenly I'm nervous to talk to her. What will she feel? The phone line crackles and we all try to talk at once.

Congratulations, I say.

No, I think I'm meant to say congratulations to you, Amanda says.

Yes, well. Congratulations anyway, that's great.

Yeah. Amanda's voice crackles. Congratulations.

I can hear that she's thrilled. Why wouldn't she be? She wants to be a surrogate mum and she wants to do it as soon as possible. Stephen and I just keep saying – Thank you and thank you and thank you. We're both staring at each other in total disbelief. How can it be that family, friends, the medical profession have been powerless to help us, and now two women in America whom we don't know have taken on our problem and are solving it for us?

Amanda explains to us that she and Manda have stayed on to visit some relatives in California. Right now they are on an island just off the coast that is famous for its frozen yoghurts. So she and Manda are going to go and have some frozen yoghurt in order to celebrate.

Frozen yoghurt, I think. Is that a good idea? Perhaps the frozen yoghurts have partly defrosted and are infested by some listeria type bug that will kill the baby? I watch my own mind running through these possibilities and I'm amazed. When I was pregnant with Thomas I ate salad and undercooked meat and never gave it a thought. And yet here I am – five and a half thousand miles away from this other woman's pregnancy – and I'm worried about what she's eating.

The call comes to an end and Stephen and I stand staring at each other.

So I'm now pregnant with a woman in a single-sex relationship in Minnesota whom I've never met, Stephen says.

No, I correct him. You're now pregnant with a nurse of Estonian origin and we don't know her name or where she lives.

Well, either way, he says, I've been getting around a bit.

We both of us feel that we should be celebrating but we don't dare. We know that a positive pregnancy test doesn't mean much. After Stephen has gone to sleep, I lie awake, crying. I'm thinking of Laura in her navy blue coat, running in that frost-glittered garden. I know now that she must be dead. And those other four babies as well. This is ridiculous, of course, but that's what I feel. She's now dead in a different and more final way than she's ever been before.

We've just embarked on the most complicated pregnancy that has ever existed. A significant number of people suffer the trauma of a stillbirth. But the combination of stillbirth, four miscarriages, failed IVF, failed adoption and then surrogacy. I've never heard of it.

It does make the Virgin Birth look fairly straightforward, Stephen says.

I'm pregnant, except that I'm not. I read on the message boards that many Intended Mothers feel jealous of their surrogate. That, at least, is one emotion I'm never going to feel. I'm very glad not to be pregnant again, thrilled that Amanda is doing this for me. But how do you prepare yourself to have a baby when you're not pregnant? I consider going to the local NCT antenatal group.

But I'm still the pregnancy leper, every woman's worst nightmare. I'm still the carrier of plague and death. I can't take myself into a room full of bright and shiny first-time mothers who are busily worrying about whether getting your hair highlighted can damage your unborn baby. I'm too old, too battered. And anyway I've always had an allergic reaction to any room which contains more than two women talking about babies.

But the question is still there. Pregnancy lasts nine months partly because it takes that long for the baby to grow, but it also lasts that long because a woman needs that time to prepare her mind for what is about to happen. But how do you create a pregnancy journey for yourself without being pregnant? And do I want to do that? I've seen plenty of pregnancies that have followed stillbirths. Inevitably they are fraught and tearful. If you've had a baby who's died then you don't make any attachment to any new baby, not until you're holding that living and breathing baby in your arms. Maybe the less I know about this pregnancy the better.

That's what I think – but I soon change my mind as the days pass and we don't hear from Amanda. I send e-mails, leave messages, but no news comes. Maybe the pregnancy has miscarried and she feels unable to tell us? I realise that I know nothing about Amanda.

I switch on the computer and call up a map of Minnesota. The state is square and to the north-west of Chicago. It is bordered by Canada to the north, the Great Lakes to the west. But where is Marshall? I press my eyes closer to the screen. Minneapolis, St Paul, Moorhead, Redwood Falls. But there is no sign of Marshall. I start to panic. Marshall does not exist. I switch the computer off and make myself busy doing other things.

And then we lose the file – the fat green file that contains everything. Everything. All my research, all the contracts we have signed, all the medical information. Everyone's address and phone number. And I've just no idea how this happened. I last saw it when Stephen and I took it to a pub in Stroud. We were having supper there and needed to discuss some papers that we were required to sign. But that was a month ago – and we've only just realised the file is missing.

We're just too casual about this. We've done it all too fast without any proper thought, as though it's just another debate with the builders about roof tiles. I search everywhere but the file never turns up. That file was all we had of our baby and now I've lost it somewhere in a pub in Stroud. It turns out that we're pretty bad at paperwork too.

I'm just about to contact Natalie, our surrogacy lawyer, to check she has copies of all the contracts when I receive an e-mail from her saying that she's moving her office from Poole to the New Forest. Fine. What does it matter? She is still going to continue to do our legal work, and confirms that she has copies of the contract. But still the move unnerves me. The world we are in is so nebulous, so abstract, that I need people to stay in the same place, I need some things to be certain. It feels as though another plank in our hastily constructed raft has gone. And still I haven't heard from Amanda in her non-existent town in the Midwest.

Then finally an e-mail arrives. Amanda is really sorry not to have been in touch but things have been complicated. She and Manda have moved house and they have both lost their jobs, although they're both hopeful that something else will come along soon. Amanda lost her job partly because she took time off to go to California for the treatment. Also Amanda no longer has her daughter, Olivia, with her because she lost custody of her. This happened because she failed to file some paperwork from the court by the required date. The move meant that the computer didn't work for a while. It will be better for them to be in town. They are close to the hospital and that's important because, when the winter comes, the roads are impassable for weeks.

I stare at the e-mail in shock. A series of assumptions I had made are fast unravelling. Amanda and Manda have a child, live in a six-bedroom house and rescue dogs. Now suddenly they're two women living in a flat in town, without the six-year-old child. And Amanda has gone from being a woman who is 'bad at paperwork' to being a woman who has lost her child because she's failed to fill out the right form.

And has Amanda really lost her job because of us? Surely that can't be right. And if she's looking for another job what kind of job will she get? Will it be a job that is suitable for a pregnant woman? Will the stress put our baby at risk? Can someone lose a job just like that? In America, they probably can. I have a row with Stephen because he just doesn't seem involved in this process. I know he's probably as scared as I am but that's no help to me. We chose to do surrogacy in America because I felt that people there are not exploited – I was wrong. I thought Amanda wasn't desperate for money – I may be wrong. I thought that this wouldn't be like reality TV but increasingly it seems to be heading that way.

The lost file, the disappearing lawyer, the town in the Midwest which doesn't exist, the unanswered calls to America, the house move, the lost jobs, the lost child. Everything is shifting all the time. There is nothing for us to have or to hold. I've spent the last six years trying to discover how you make the absent present, but I still don't know how to do it. Before, I was trying to give life to a person who no one could see. Now I'm trying to give life to another person we can't see.

I'd like to sit down and cry but I can't do that because somewhere, unseen, in the middle of this mess, there's a person who is now perhaps three or four centimetres long, a person swimming in a sack of fluid in that non-existent town. She may be four thousand miles away but we were responsible for bringing her into existence so now we have to look after her. I find Stephen in his study and we talk about what we're going to do. We're both trying to pretend that we're not too worried. We call IARC and they promise to call back in an hour.

As I put the washing machine on, hang clothes on the line, load the dishwasher, I realise how incredibly grateful I am to have IARC on our side. I know from websites that some people try to do surrogacy without an agency. I can't imagine how they manage that. I couldn't possibly have any kind of business conversation with Amanda. I couldn't point out a clause in a contract to her or argue over what we are and aren't going to pay. She is carrying my husband's child so I have to get on with her.

IARC are not concerned. It soon becomes apparent that in America people lose their jobs all the time because they have no employment protection. We ask IARC if we should pay Amanda not to go back to work. They tell us that contractually we have no obligation to do that but agree that it might ease the situation.

After we put the phone down I say to Stephen – What do you reckon? Should we pay?

Oh yes, he says. Of course we should pay. There's no question about that. If you were pregnant and I thought you shouldn't be working I wouldn't let you – so of course we should do the same for Amanda. But that isn't the issue.

He's sitting at his desk in legal mode.

The problem is, he says, that when we come back to the UK we have to go to the High Court and show that we haven't paid more than 'reasonable expenses'. What I don't know is whether this would be a 'reasonable expense'.

We should ask Natalie, I say.

No, he says. Because if she says we shouldn't do it, then later we would have to admit to having gone against her advice. We'll just do it and deal with the consequences later.

Are you sure?

Yes, I'm sure. I'll ring IARC and sort it.

Soon we have an e-mail from Amanda. She's incredibly grateful for the money and the situation is easier because Manda has two new jobs now. Also, she's just been for a twelve week scan and our baby had a heartbeat. She wants to know what we will call her. I stall, say that we're thinking about it and will get back to her.

But a week later Amanda raises the issue again. Clearly it's important to her and to Manda that this person who is living with them should have a name. I ask Stephen what he thinks. He doesn't really want to discuss this question because, for him, it's tempting fate. He just can't bear any more disappointment but I'm full of confidence.

Although I worry about everything, strangely I never really worry about our baby. And that's because I know that Amanda is looking after her just fine. I wasn't confident with any of the last four pregnancies. I knew they would fail and I knew the IVF would result in nothing. And yet I know this will work. But I can't choose a name on my own.

Perhaps we should go for a temporary name? Often couples have a nickname for their unborn child. We can't call our child The Bump because we haven't seen any bump. Thomas was called The Wriggler because he wriggled so much. We're never going to know whether this baby wriggles or not. So what can we do?

And then, out of nowhere, a name arrives – Hope. That's her name because that's what she represents to us. Except that this idea is so sentimental that it embarrasses me. So I try to lay it aside, laugh it off, shut it out of the door. But it refuses to be shifted, clings on tight. Hope is the name she has to have. The matter seems to have been decided whether I'm in agreement or not.

Of course, the Black Humour Department of my brain points out that, should she die, then that will be The Death of Hope. But then that is what it will be – literally and meta-phorically – so that at least satisfies the writerly part of me, which insists that things must be called by their proper names. At least for the moment, we have Hope.

One day I pick Thomas up from school and he tells me that he has been learning about the parable of the Good Samaritan. I should just take the conventional line, tell him that the Good Samaritan is an important role model. But the problem is that I myself have been thinking of that parable recently – and questioning the assumptions that lie behind it. I've been think-ing of Joslin's skill in avoiding people at the hospice when the need arises. Ever since Laura died, I've been on a mission to look after the depressed and the suffering. In endless support groups, I have held the hands of weeping bereaved mothers. On the phone late at night I've listened to their stories without ever dwelling on mine. But what good have I really done? And what has been the result for me? In truth, I am tired out by goodness.

I don't know, I say to Thomas. Maybe after two thousand years of disapproval the Pharisee is ripe for reappraisal? Maybe we haven't been entirely fair on him? I mean, it never actually says why he did that, does it? Maybe he'd already picked up five other wounded men that day? Perhaps he was on his way to his elderly mother's ninetieth birthday party and was already two hours late?

After this school-run conversation, I decide to stop being good. It's time for me to realise that, in order to cope with Laura's death, I don't have to put a splint on every lame duck that I meet. And strangely I feel much better. I am puzzled. The equation is meant to be: goodness equals happiness. Lack of compassion equals unhappiness. But in reality the equation doesn't really seem to work that way.

Spring arrives like an overenthusiastic visitor, bringing warmth, green, a sudden slowing of the days. I should be glad but it's all too much for me, I am horribly tired all the time. I realise that I'm struggling even to climb a normal staircase. I go to the doctor and discover that I'm anaemic. This shouldn't be the case as I'm already taking iron pills. One day, in an attempt to raise my energy levels, I eat a huge lunch of sausage, chips, beans, milky coffee. I haven't eaten like this in years because I've been trying to look after my health by eating lots of salad and vegetables. But after lunch I feel so much better that I am forced to the conclusion that healthy eating is bad for my health. Another equation which shouldn't work out – but does.

Amanda goes for her fifteen week scan and we wait for news. She e-mails to say that she didn't actually see Hope but she heard her heartbeat. She tried to make a video recording of the heartbeat and she's going to send it to us. I'm not quite sure what this means. A couple of days later Amanda e-mails to say that unfortunately she can't make it work. When she tried to transfer the recording to her computer, the sound didn't come through and so she's decided not to send it.

Probably a good decision, I think. A recording of a heartbeat without the sound is probably not a meaningful experience. When I discuss this with Stephen we both start laughing and can't stop. All of this seems symptomatic of this weird world we are in. The truth is that we don't really want to hear the heartbeat because we've heard too many heartbeats that have stopped.

XXIV

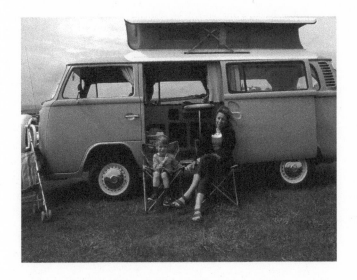

Never apologise for showing feeling.
When you do so, you apologise for the truth.

Benjamin Disraeli

I don't speak to anyone about what really frightens me. The birth itself. I have never been near a newborn baby since Laura died. Will I want to hold Hope? I hear the voices of those women in the support group. *I can't touch him, I can't look at him. He's the wrong baby. The wrong baby.*

Will Hope be the wrong baby? Will I ever believe that she's going to stay alive, that she's going to keep on breathing? I just don't know. When I think of the hospital, the birth, a new baby, tiny, dark red, wrinkled, screaming. Blood, pain. A baby which is so warm to the touch but dead, totally and completely dead. My mind closes down.

I speak to my mum and she says that she'll come with us to America. But Mum has never liked going far from home and she's now seventy-three. She knows that, in reality, she might be more of a hindrance than a help. I tell Stephen that I'm worried about how we're going to cope in America. There will be so many relationships to be managed, so many legal issues to sort. What if I'm ill or if the baby is ill? What if I have to stay in America on my own with the baby? In a hotel room, in a city where I know no one. I'm just not in a state where I would be able to do that. Together Stephen and I agree that we need to find someone to go with us to America.

Then I remember a smart West London friend who had a maternity nurse – someone to look after her and the baby immediately after the birth. I look up agencies online, make phone calls and find out more. The agencies send CVs. We interview a couple of people and are uncertain whether they might be the right person or not. And then a CV comes for a woman called Linda McKinnon. She lives in France and lists her hobbies as yoga, organic food and cycling. She's worked before for a family with a surrogate baby. And so, one evening, sitting on the big sofa in the playroom, I give her a call.

Immediately I like her voice and so I make an arrangement for her to meet Stephen and me in London. Lin is tall, tanned and elegant with scatty-looking hair and lozenge-shaped horn-rimmed glasses. Her CV says that she's sixty but she could pass for fifty. She is full of confidence about our trip to America. She has travelled with many families and their babies. Nothing will be a problem. She will help out with Thomas as well. All we have to do is to call when Hope is on the way and she can be with us in a few hours. As soon as Lin leaves, Stephen and I agree that we will offer her the job and I feel less frightened. If I can't cope with the baby, then Lin will cope until I recover my sanity.

IARC get in touch to say that all the legal arrangements are now in place and that we can get in touch with our egg donor directly. Her name is Elena and she lives in North Dakota. I hesitate, wondering what sort of message might be appropriate to our situation.

It's the weekend of the Royal Wedding. It's also Joslin's birthday and I should have gone but I haven't. Instead I'm at my mum's farm, sitting at the kitchen table, checking my e-mails, when a message arrives from Elena. I take several deep breaths and open it, read hurriedly. Elena has got in touch because she wants to tell us a little more of her story.

She married young, she says, and she always knew that she wanted a family, but she and her husband waited several years and she never got pregnant. Eventually they went for tests. They expected to receive the results over the phone but instead they were asked to go into the clinic. There they were told that Elena had a problem with her tubes. It is likely, the medical staff told her, that you will never have a child of your own.

But still they offered to try IVF and against all the odds Elena got pregnant with triplets. Obviously it was a high-risk pregnancy but all three babies – Melissa, Carrie and Edward – were born in good health. Once they were four years old Elena decided to become an egg donor. She needed some money because triplets are expensive, but she also knew that she was the ideal person to be an egg donor because she had finished having her own family young and, also, as a nurse she wasn't unnerved by the medical procedures involved.

But that wasn't all. In her e-mail she writes – I also knew that I wanted to do it because I've never forgotten that moment at the clinic when they said I'd never be able to have a child of my own. I always remember what that felt like and so to me it's very important to donate eggs. It's a way of acknowledging how lucky I am.

Elena has attached some photographs of her triplets to the e-mail. I know that these children are now eight years old but I've only ever seen one small, blurred photograph of them when they were two. These children are Hope's half siblings. I'm frightened to open the attachment. What if I look at these children and there is something about them that simply doesn't appeal? The internet connection is slow and it takes hours for the photographs to open. I sit staring at small blocks advancing across the screen. Thomas is telling me a long story about a dog, a stick, a water trough and a catapult.

Then suddenly a photograph appears. It shows three children – two girls and a boy – at a Thanksgiving party, wearing their best clothes. The girls' dresses are shiny blue satin and the boy wears a beige shirt and chinos. And they're stunning, simply stunning – in a way that I hadn't expected at all. They look Polish to me, East European. For some reason their pale perfection makes me think of photographs of American pioneer families. I can't stop staring at them. I take the computer and run across the yard to where my mum is washing down a pony. She stops and comes to look. Neither of us have anything to say. Suddenly all this is real because these are the half siblings of my daughter.

But I'm embarrassed as well. All those headlines about designer babies come back to me. I didn't need a beautiful, blonde little girl. Any little girl would have done. But still I'm amazed and excited. And the main thing is that these children could be mine. They look a bit like me. For ages afterwards my mind bounces from one thought to another crazily. It's too much to take in.

My mum takes Thomas out for a ride down the lane on a tiny pony called Maxwell. I lag behind them, walking slowly, so that they arrive back at the farm before me. Then Thomas comes running back up the road towards me. He wants to go and see Laura's grave. I have already been once but now he wants to go as well. He collects daisies and buttercups and lays them out in an intricate pattern on the grave. The grass is dry so we sit down. Thomas talks about dead people not being comfortable in their graves and suddenly we're laughing about imaginary complaints – *this coffin is too small, it's badly ventilated, my feet are cold.*

I wonder what Laura actually is now. Possibly the clothes she was buried in have lasted better than her flesh. But what clothes was she buried in? The truth is I don't know. The hospital should have offered me the opportunity to dress her in whatever I wanted. I should also have put my grandmother's ring on a ribbon around her neck. I suspect that she is just a bit of dust and some tiny bones now – something like a chicken carcass that has been picked clean. She would have been six in May.

Joslin is having chemotherapy again and has to go to Hereford Hospital every Tuesday. I try and meet her there when I can because it's easier to drive to Hereford than Hay-on-Wye. I'll be in the Charles Renton Unit, she says. The name sounds encouraging, but the unit turns out to be a row of Nissen huts at the back of the hospital, a forgotten corner of the NHS.

As I'm parking, I catch sight of Joslin. But is that her? Her hair had come back briefly but now it's gone again. Her scalp is luminous white, her face slightly tanned. She wears a back brace, walks with a stick, has grown bigger. I only recognise her because I know the patchwork cardigan and remember the bag that we bought together in Hereford at Christmas.

The nurses in the Chemotherapy Unit wear too much make-up and are relentlessly cheerful. They insist that everyone is getting on just fine. But who can blame them? Doing this work day to day – how else can they cope? Again we're in the hairdressing salon for people with no hair. The machines bing-bing-bing cheerfully. The patients are neatly contained within their own silent stories. The obvious questions are not asked.

After Joslin has had her treatment we agree to go over to the main hospital for a coffee. It takes me a while to find a wheelchair and the one that I find is fantastically badly designed. It is heavy and uncontrollable so that we weave dangerously from one side of the hospital corridor to the other. It should take five minutes to reach the canteen but instead it takes fifteen. The coffee shop is near the hospital entrance and has plate-glass windows that look out over the forecourt. The chairs are pine coloured with narrow waists. As I bring a coffee for Joslin, a woman approaches us. She says that she wants to talk to Joslin and would it be all right for her to sit down? Of course, we agree, although I'm concerned that this might not be the right thing for Joslin. She shouldn't have to cope with anyone else's problems when her own is surely the greatest tragedy of them all.

The woman who sits down with us is elderly, with soft grey-black hair. She wears a silk shirt, tailored trousers, a wool cardigan which coordinates with the shirt. Her glasses hang from a gold chain around her neck. Despite her age, the skin of her face is soft and, although she has dark shadows under her eyes, those eyes are lively and deep-diving.

It is Joslin, isn't it? I was sure I recognised you. You are Joslin, aren't you?

Clearly she recognises Joslin from some other corner of Cancer World – Cheltenham Hospital perhaps? Joslin seems uncertain if she recognises the woman or not. Presumably she has met many people on her long travels around the Oncology Centres and the Chemotherapy Units.

You had a baby, didn't you? the woman says.

She wants to ask about the health of the baby and Joslin explains that Lily is now nearly two. And Ellie and James are six and seven.

So how is the treatment going? The woman asks. This question is not normally asked. Joslin says that the treatment is all right.

But you've had to have more treatment?

Again I wonder if we've made a mistake in starting this conversation.

I got breast cancer three years ago, the woman says. And

I had a double mastectomy but now I'm back again. I don't think they know what to do with me. I've just been for another scan and now I'm waiting for the results.

She shrugs and then says – But then I am seventy-eight.

This comes as a surprise because she could pass for ten years younger.

Suddenly Joslin is awake, passionate. Yes, she says. Yes. But you still want your life. Everyone wants their life. It doesn't matter what age you are. You still want your life.

The truth of this hits me coldly. With the callousness of the relatively young, I tend to assume that once you reach a certain age then you've had your innings, that you must know you haven't got long.

Yes, the woman agrees. And then she tells us her name. Jennifer Williams.

And so we introduce ourselves – Alice and Joslin.

I hope you don't mind that I disturbed you, she said. I just wanted you to know, and so now perhaps when you see me around you'll say hello.

Joslin says she certainly will, but explains that she's dosed full of morphine and so often forgets. Jennifer agrees the morphine is a problem. She can often hardly remember anything at all.

So just tell me, Joslin says. If I don't notice you, then just come up to me and say – Hello, I'm Alice.

Jennifer lays a hand gently on Joslin's arm. I'm called Jennifer.

All three of us laugh.

Ah well. I must be going, Jennifer says. But you will remember, won't you?

Yes, we say.

If you see me around you will remember, won't you? Jennifer Williams.

Yes.

So if you're passing.

Yes.

And so she disappears, weaving away around a distant corner, her glasses swinging from her chain. I'm looking forward to a moment of peace with Joslin but Terry appears. He has come to drive Joslin home. I've met Terry before, he is a volunteer for a local cancer charity. His wife died of cancer a year ago. He told me that when we first met.

We had such fantastic support, he says. I had to put something back.

Terry is now trying to help Joslin get into the car – although it is questionable whether he is any more able-bodied than she is. I help them both, thank Terry.

S'right, he says. Then he nods in the direction of Joslin. It's a privilege to drive this one. A real privilege.

I am left on the hospital forecourt, aching. And all the way home I think of Terry and his dead wife, the courage which he must need to get up in the morning and drive cancer victims back and forth to the hospital. And I think of Jennifer Williams who still wants her life. You will remember, won't you? I'm Jennifer Williams. You will remember, won't you? Jennifer Williams.

We haven't told Thomas yet about Hope but we know we will have to do it soon. I dread the moment. How can we possibly explain all this to a nine-year-old? In June we are going to Cornwall for a week and Stephen and I agree that we'll tell him then. We travel around Cornwall in a hired mustard-coloured VW camper van called Sheila and then meet up with my mum and spend a few days at the Nare Hotel on the south coast, looking out over the sea. Stephen and I disagree about where we should have our conversation with Thomas. I think we should discuss it at breakfast. Stephen worries about other guests overhearing and favours the beach.

And so there we are, sitting in a circle of rocks, pulling our swimming things from bags. And we say to Thomas that we have something important to tell him. Then he is wailing, flapping his arms up and down, trying to bury his face in the nearest rock. His small feet kick at the sand, his mouth spits. He doesn't want a baby sister. He hates babies. He likes being an only child. And why, why, why did we have to tell him like this? When he's on the beach having fun?

Oddly he is entirely uninterested in surrogacy, in America, in all things to do with the origins of this baby. Instead he stands, skinny and tearful in his swimming trunks, his face wobbling, still kicking at the sand, and talks about territory. This baby will steal his Lego and tear his books. He will never let her into his room, never. She will not be allowed to share any of his toys, ever.

Stephen and I point out that it will be years before she has even the smallest interest in his toys. I try to take him in my arms but he pushes me away. The day, which was warm, now seems surprisingly chilly. I pull my jumper back on over my swimsuit, try not to cry. Mum insists that Thomas should go down to the sea with her and reluctantly he goes. I watch the two of them, far down the beach, holding hands, jumping over waves. Stephen and I look at each other, shrug. I set off back up to the hotel.

I know that Thomas is entitled to his own reaction to our news. But I needed him to be pleased, to offer his support. I'm frightened that we've made a terrible mistake. By trying to have something more, we have wrecked what we already have. That circle of rocks, Thomas's angry screams, the cooling sky. That's a day on the beach I would love to forget.

XXV

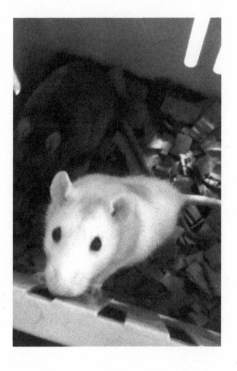

Speak properly, and in as few words as you can, but plainly;
for the end of speech is not ostentation,
but to be understood.

William Penn

Natalie gets in touch to say that she needs that twenty-page statement explaining everything that led us to surrogacy in America. This is part of our preparation for the hearing in the High Court where it will be decided whether we will be granted a Parental Order. I intend to respond but days pass and I do nothing. It's all there in the cardboard box in my study but why look at it? I prefer to enjoy my non-existent existence.

Two weeks later Natalie e-mails again to ask how I'm getting on. I give myself a firm talking to, then pull that box out of the cupboard. There it is – the last five years of my life. Breathe, remember to breathe. A ragged pile of diaries, photos, e-mails, blog entries, sentences scrawled in notebooks. A memoir which I never intended to write. But how can I organise it? I have no idea how the jigsaw of days and months fits together.

It's like when you play the piano and your left hand stretches down to a low note, a distant C, but it doesn't make the sound that it should. Instead the thread of your melody breaks up in a discordant clanking. All I need to do is to establish the chronology, to ensure that when I stretch my mind back through the past, I find the notes of my keyboard where they should properly be.

I sit down and provide the barrister with the information she needs – more or less – although I still can't find that missing year. Once I've done that I could put the cardboard box away and try to forget. But instead I find myself still writing, trying to settle the ghosts more comfortably in their graves. *This coffin is too small, it's badly ventilated, my feet are cold.*

When psychiatrists try to treat victims of trauma one of the techniques they use is to make the victim repeat his or her story again and again. This is meant to help with the processing of grief. Now I write and rewrite, again and again. Lay the world out in long, straight rows of black on white, word after word, neat and orderly. A book has boundaries, edges, it comes to an end. It is like a box, its cover a lid. You can open it when you want to – and shut it as well. I'm trying to find a way to maintain my love for one child, while making space for another. And I'm writing to keep myself sane. I write because I cannot speak.

Deep down, all the time, is the fear that Amanda will want to keep our baby. The agency tell me that they have organised hundreds of surrogate births and they've never seen this problem. In America the law relating to gestational surrogacy is clear. If a surrogate mother tries to keep the baby then the law will not be on her side.

I don't find this comforting. If you have to wrestle a baby from another woman's arms then the fact that you might succeed won't count for much. I know what it feels like to leave hospital without the baby you carried, but this is not the same. Amanda wants to do this.

But still I'm worried. I talk to Keely at the agency about how things will be managed at the hospital. She says that no one from the agency will be there but that, should any abnormal behaviour arise, then I should report it to the agency immediately. But in this surreal world how will I know what constitutes abnormal?

I get an e-mail from Amanda which says that she's really going to find life flat and boring once the surrogacy is over and Hope has gone home. My she's-going-to-keep-my-baby antennae fizz. But then I realise that I need to listen at a deeper level.

Through my research I know that one of the problems that a surrogate mother faces is that, afterwards, she can never say – I feel really down. Because everyone immediately thinks that she wanted to keep the baby. But she can feel sad without regretting her decision. Everyone has the Baby Blues, no matter what the circumstances.

What do I need to do to help Amanda through this? We can't just jet in and take Hope away. We're going to have to find a balance between letting Amanda show her love for Hope but not letting her feel that essential bond of motherhood. We're in this together, I owe her everything and I'm going to have to find ways to make this as easy as possible. But I don't know how.

I now have a strong sense of Hope. Of course, there's no way I can have a sense of her. She's four thousand miles away and she isn't genetically my daughter. But still I know her. Strangely, what I feel is a strong link between her and my mother. Hope is a farm girl: strong, practical, balanced. A girl with her sleeves rolled up and an admirable lack of patience with the abstract or theoretical. She's tougher than Thomas, tougher than me.

Like my mother, she doesn't say much but she knows. She's patient and constant, a girl who has no question about the way things are but gets on with the day cheerfully. Her genes have travelled from Estonia to America, and now will travel back to Gloucestershire in England. She's already ancient and so she's rooted and calm in the way that Thomas and I are not.

Of course, all of this is total invention, dangerous invention. Hope is already a baby with a history so she doesn't need me to create a future for her as well. But still the knowledge persists. I know her, I just do. Pregnancy is not only a physical journey but also a mental one – and it turns out that the mental aspects of it develop anyway even when the physical pregnancy is so many miles away.

Thomas seems happier now about the idea of a baby sister but I need to look after him, to make sure he feels included. So when he asks for a hamster, yet again, I decide that I can no longer avoid the rodent road. I make various enquiries and we are on the point of getting a hamster when, by chance, I meet a woman who has three hundred rats. She is called Jacky and she runs a rat rescue organisation which is called Rat Out Of Hell.

Oh. Right. So how do you find out about rats that need rescuing?

There's a very big online rat community.

Uuum. Yeah. I suppose there would be. And these rats – I mean, are they like the ones under the floorboards?

Clearly I've asked the wrong question. Jacky's rats are fancy rats and have nothing to do with floorboards, apparently. Before I know it, I have offered to let her provide me with two for Thomas. And so Sergei and Alexander become part of our family. The first time that Thomas lets them out of the cage they hide in the base of the sofa and it takes us two hours to get them out. I don't touch them but Thomas spends hours cuddling them and allowing them to run across his arms and shoulders, sitting them on his head.

I am morbidly sensitive about what other people will say when they find out about the surrogacy, what judgements they will make. I'm endlessly waiting for someone to express their disapproval. I probe this fear. What exactly is it? I fear their disapproval not because I can't understand it but because I understand it only too well. We only ever find ourselves in conflict with people with whom we share common ground. I know that. But it's too late. We're doing it now.

And we have to start telling people. We start with family and move on from there. Everyone says exactly the same – Oh I knew. I just knew. Because recently you've just had that special glow about you. You know, like people have when they're pregnant?

I tell people at the Nailsworth Quaker Meeting House and they receive the news with excitement and enthusiasm, an absolute lack of judgement. I say – Don't you worry about the morality of this?

I am told that people have trust in me and my judgement. If I think that this is the right thing for me to do, then it's right.

Mothers at the school are shocked but supportive. Stephen says – I have a feeling we'll be filling the gap between the cheese and the coffee at Gloucestershire dinner parties for weeks to come.

One day I am telling one of the mothers at school when a little girl called Lotte walks past. The next day at school Lotte lets it be known that she knows a secret about Thomas. She's asked by all the children exactly what she heard.

Thomas is soon going to be getting a small snake, she says.

Thomas's status soars. Not only is he the owner of two rats, but soon he will also be the proud possessor of a small snake. Even after Lotte admits to having invented the snake, the idea of it still slithers around the school, bringing with it delight and terror and confusion. And what with the actual rats and the anticipated small snake, Hope becomes irrelevant. Who cares about baby sisters? Everyone has one of those, all they do is steal your Lego.

Finally, the only person who is nasty about the surrogacy is a woman whom I know through the stillbirth support group. She is someone that I offered to help for no reason other than that I was terribly sorry about the death of her fourth child, a baby son. But now that I need her, she doesn't even bother to hear the whole story, but jumps in with criticism and condemnation.

Ah well, no good turn goes unpunished. I don't mind her criticism but I'm angry that she didn't even bother to establish the basic facts before forcing her opinions on me. I know I should rise above the situation, feel compassion rather than disappointment. But I'm bored with seeing other people's point of view and decide that I'd rather indulge in some good old-fashioned hatred.

Every few weeks an insurmountable legal problem occurs. We are living in an elevator which is running out of control. It whizzes up and down randomly. Our stomachs are left hanging, pressed up into our mouths. We don't get time to catch our breath before it drops again. The latest problem is that the US courts need evidence that Stephen and I are good citizens with no criminal convictions. The UK courts will also need this evidence, but the Court Reporter will ask for it when we are back in the UK. The problem is that the Americans need this information soon after the birth. So how can that be solved?

I could worry about all this but I don't. Hope is alive and

well and we're going to bring her home. We'll do it somehow, it will happen. The legal stuff is irrelevant. I sign forms, get them witnessed, send them off. Stephen talks to the lawyers and I ignore the issue. I remember when I was pregnant with Thomas, during the last three months, I was filled with a wonderful calm. I talked to more experienced mothers who said – Oh yes, of course, the la-la-la-la hormone, everyone gets that late in pregnancy. Maybe that's what I'm getting now even though I'm not pregnant.

On the phone to Natalie I say – Listen, I just don't see why this has to be so complicated. I mean, what usually happens? We're not the first people who have ever done this so how does it normally work?

The phone is silent. Then a slight sound of a throat clearing.

Um. Yes, actually you are.

What?

The first people to bring a surrogate baby home from the state of Minnesota.

Oh. Right. I'm glad I didn't find this out sooner.

After we've put the phone down, I say to Stephen – Are you really sure we need to do all of this? Don't you think we might be OK if we just walked through Heathrow and hoped for the best?

But Stephen is adamant. This can be done within the law and it will be.

I wonder what it will mean to Hope to be both a surrogate baby and donor conceived. It may be unsettling to know that another woman carried you through pregnancy, but still it is the donor question that is most complicated. Online I find an organisation called the Donor Conception Network and learn that nearly two thousand babies are now born in the UK each year from donor eggs, donor sperm or donor embryos.

The DCN is a national organisation of parents of donor conceived children. A conference is taking place in a school on the outskirts of Bristol and I sign up. As I approach the entrance to the school, I am surrounded by others heading in the same direction, couples, single women, children. I look at the children and think – so is that child genetically linked to that father, that mother? I have never before had cause to ask a question of this kind.

Once in the spacious entrance hall, the situation becomes even more awkward. We have all come here for one reason and one reason only, but the details that lie behind all the stories amassing here are deeply personal, not questions you discuss with strangers. But then why come if you're not going to talk? I find myself a cup of tea, hover. A woman who is clearly one of the organisers appears and I ask her if there are any other people at the conference with surrogate babies. Apparently among the two hundred people attending I am the only one. Ah well.

But then a woman steps forward, introduces herself and dives straight in. Her name is Rachel and she is a single mum with a daughter who is eighteen and a son who is six. She got married young, had her daughter, but then, when she was thirty-nine, her marriage broke up. She didn't mind about the marriage but she minded desperately that she would never have another child. And so she decided to go it alone. There's a book, she says. It's called *How to Get Yourself Knocked Up – A Single Woman's Guide to Pregnancy*.

Oh. Right. Yes.

The Czech Republic, she tells me. That's where you go. Under the system there you never know the identity of the donor. Mainly they are university students wanting to make some money. For me, at a conference like this it's weird because I look around at the children and wonder if any of them are related to my son.

Rachel lives in a small village in Staffordshire and when she got pregnant people did want to know who the father was. But overall everyone has been surprisingly supportive and open-minded. She knows that one day her son will be angry with her. I'll just have to do the best I can when that moment comes, she says.

Privately I am inevitably asking the question which everyone must ask. Should she have been allowed to do what she did? I am hardly in a position to judge. She could have just had a one-night stand and forgotten the man's name. The result would have been the same but perhaps the approach she took was more honest?

We are joined by a man who has two sons conceived using donor sperm. He cheerfully suggests that the importance of a genetic link is vastly overestimated. In my family, he says, we have jug ears, flat feet and occasional schizophrenia. I'm very happy not to see any of those characteristics repeated in my sons.

As I go to get myself a second cup of tea, I meet Evan who tells me that he is an Altruistic Sperm Donor.

Oh, right, I say. Great. Lovely. Well, um. So-o-o-o?

I just give people sperm for free, he says.

I wonder if we're talking about one-night stands or the turkey baster.

So do you have children yourself? I ask.

No, he says. I never wanted them. But there are now seventeen children who were conceived using my sperm. Some of the mothers are single, some lesbian, some married.

Oh right. That's wonderful. So do you see the children?

Well, yeah. Some more than others. It was one of the lesbian couples who asked me to come along today. Just thought I'd find out what it's all about. Of course, I sign a legal agreement to make sure I can't be asked to pay child support. I'm happy to meet any of the children any time. I wish them all well.

So why? I ask. What made you decide to do this?

Well, the thing is that I'm a really great guy. I'm good-looking and I'm clever and I'm also a nice bloke.

The annoying thing about this statement is that it's clearly true.

So anyway, he says. I just feel that my seed should be widely scattered, that the world would be a better place if there were more people like me in it.

Evan raises an eyebrow, gives me a quizzical smile, and is swept away by a crowd of people heading towards the sports hall for the main session of the conference.

Everyone who speaks in these sessions stresses the importance of being totally honest with children about their origins. But when the conference breaks into smaller groups different views emerge. Who owns the information? Who has the right to decide who is told? Interesting distinctions are drawn between secrecy and privacy. Someone asks what, in this world of new technology, the word mother means? She is told that a mother is the person who does the mothering but I am unsure if it's really that simple.

One woman who is pregnant with a donor embryo child says – If you received a kidney from a donor you wouldn't want to know about that person, would you? It is pointed out to her – gently – that a kidney is not the same as genetic material. And that finally is the nub of the question. It all comes down to the ancient nature–nurture debate. The question of identity, of what makes us into the people that we are.

On the train home, I turn all the questions of the day over in my head. Most of us do think about our genetic heritage often. We use it to explain aspects of our lives. *I like the countryside because my mother likes the countryside. I hate maths because my father hated maths.* We use statements such as these as markers, as guides, as a means to navigate through the confusion of life. We use them to explain who we are and why we make the choices that we make.

But the interesting thing is that there is no scientific certainty to such statements. *I like the countryside because my mother likes the countryside.* In truth there could be three possible reasons why this statement is true. Genetics might be the explanation, but this preference might also be explained by environmental factors. Or it may be nothing more than coincidence.

These statements that we make are merely stories that we tell, picking out the facts that fit a narrative which we've already created. After all, it is true that my mother and I both like the countryside, but I have neglected to note that she has brown hair and I am blonde.

But what of the donor conceived child? Genetic heritage may be nothing more than narrative but that doesn't mean it has no importance. The problem for the donor conceived child is that the narrative is harder to create because some of the landmarks are missing. But Hope will know about Elena. She will be able to ask – are there people in your family who love music? She will be able to recognise a chin or an eyebrow that will allow her to fit her own face into a lineage of faces. Will that be enough to anchor her? I can only hope that it will.

July arrives and we set off for Cornwall, stay in the Carbis Bay Hotel, just outside St Ives. One evening, at 10.15, we're scheduled to receive a call from America. Amanda will make the call from her hospital appointment and we're expecting to speak to Dr Hartfiel, who is going to deliver Hope, as well as to Amanda herself. But it isn't going to be easy for Stephen and me to manage the call because mobile reception in this area is poor and who will look after Thomas?

I suggest that we use the landline in the hotel bedroom but it doesn't have a speaker phone so we won't both be able to listen. Stephen works out that we can get mobile reception if we stand out in the garden of the hotel, at the end of the swimming pool. That will mean leaving Thomas alone in the hotel room but he will be able to wave from the window if he needs us.

So we agree on the swimming pool plan. Day turns to night – one of those balmy, Cornish evenings of bitter, rattling rain. A lively wind is blowing in from the sea, tearing at palm trees and striped awnings. But still at ten o'clock Stephen and I head out and sit by the pool, on sun loungers, sheltered by dripping sun umbrellas. Steam rises off the turquoise pool and a smell of chlorine pinches our noses.

Up above us we can see the lights of the hotel, the shadows of other people at the windows, getting ready for bed. A train rumbles past on the line that runs above the hotel gardens, the surf breaks on the beach below. Occasionally the sun umbrellas are caught by a gust of wind and deposit buckets of water all around us. Beyond the hotel, the lights of Carbis Bay stretch away in a crescent, glittering in the darkness.

The call doesn't come and it doesn't come. Stephen tries to ring and doesn't get through. He sends an e-mail and a text. Thomas appears on the balcony of our room and so I head up the bank towards the hotel to find out what is wrong. He's only asking when we'll come back in but, while I'm dealing with him, Stephen gestures furiously to let me know that the call has come.

Amanda, Manda, Dr Hartfiel and Keely in Minnesota are all on the call. Everyone talks at once in a confusion of enthusiasm and goodwill. We're asked what we want for the birth and it is suggested that we might draw up a birth plan. I'm grateful that we're being asked, but I don't really see what right I have to tell another woman how to give birth.

I'm not planning to have any drugs in the labour, Amanda says.

That's great, I say. That's fine. But you can have whatever you want.

And that's what we say again and again – whatever is good for Amanda will be good for us. Then Dr Hartfiel asks if we would like to hear the heartbeat and suddenly it's there, incredibly strong and fast, like a galloping horse. A pounding rhythm which comes to us with three-dimensional clarity from four thousand miles across the Atlantic. The sound is powerful and will never come to an end.

Stephen and I are sitting there grabbing tight to each other's hand. Suddenly a great gust of wind comes in off the sea, hits the umbrella above and dumps a bucket of freezing rainwater all over us so that Stephen has to shake the water out of the phone and we don't know whether the liquid running down our cheeks is rain or tears.

And Hope is still with us, a galloping horse enclosed in the black plastic square of Stephen's mobile phone. She's moving at incredible speed, strong and confident with mane waving and hooves pounding. And she's heading towards us across all that vast night and all the salty blackness of that great sea. Coming to us in Carbis Bay, St Ives. Coming home.

XXVI

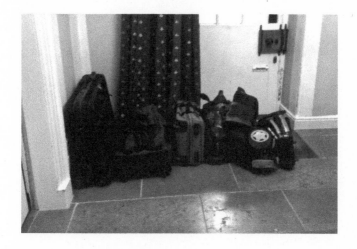

Not everything that is faced can be changed,
but nothing can be changed until it is faced.

James Baldwin

August. Riots break out in London. In Libya the National Transitional Council takes control of Tripoli and forces Gaddafi from power. It's two months now until we go to America. I get a text saying that Joslin's condition is worse and she won't leave the hospice again. I stare at the phone, unable to absorb this information. I'd assumed that Joslin had at least six months to live. She wants so much to be alive to see Hope but that's not going to happen now.

I'm at the farm with my mum and Thomas when this news comes. Mum offers to look after Thomas and so I set off for the hospice, driving the dipping and winding road that leads to Ledbury and then on towards Hereford. The morning is bright but fast-moving clouds are rushing across the sky – the kind that suddenly cast dappled shadows across the landscape. And the shadows seem longer and darker than they should be. I play music loudly, try not to think.

I've no idea what I will find at the hospice. Wayland has told me that Joslin is only able to speak a few words occasionally so I don't know whether she'll be conscious, or even if I'll be able to see her. But as it turns out, I'm able to go straight into her room. She lies twisted up by the pain, pale and swollen, her head covered with the faintest fuzz of pale hair. Without eyebrows, her face is a dull moon.

I know what they're doing, she says. They want me to see the children now in case I don't see them again. How dare they suggest that? She gasps with pain, her voice pleads. I'm not ready to die. I'm very scared.

Her room at the hospice is not the same room as she had before but it nevertheless looks out over the same view – an average bit of Herefordshire countryside but attractive all the same, and possessing an added resonance, because it must have been viewed by so many who are dying. Today we see small fruit trees in regimental rows and the unchanging hills, a formless shape, behind.

I've seen robins and pigeons, Joslin says. And squirrels. I like the squirrels.

She wants some fruit although she already has some.

I haven't eaten anything since I got here ten days ago, she says.

She's only actually been in the hospice for five days. I know she's desperately hungry but she can't eat. Together we make a list of food she thinks she might be able to manage – fruit, yoghurt, juice – and I agree to go to Hereford to get it. I know she won't be able to eat any of the fruit but that isn't the point.

I'm in pain everywhere, she says. I'm bleeding everywhere.

I don't really understand this, but as I'm leaving I speak to a male nurse who confirms that it's true. She's peeing blood, shitting it, vomiting it. I ask the nurse how long she's got. He says she might have a few days – or maybe weeks. I drive to Hereford and get the fruit. When I come back Joslin is either sleeping or unconscious. I want her to die now because I don't want her to be in pain any more.

I leave my number with the nurses and ask them to call if the situation gets worse. I decide that I won't go back tomorrow but maybe I'll go on Wednesday. Deep down, as I drive away from the hospice through the Herefordshire countryside, which is somehow autumnal even though it's still summer, a nasty little voice inside me says – *Thank God it isn't me.*

I buy a map of the state of Minnesota. In some nightmare corner of my mind, I still suspect that Marshall doesn't exist. I lay the map out on the playroom floor. I find the County of Marshall but I've already been warned that the county and the town are not the same place. Finally I find the town, a tiny dot on the map, identified by writing almost too small to read. I show it to Thomas.

Oh no, he says. Look, it's right near Springfield. You know, the Simpsons. Is our baby going to be small and yellow with a thing like a rubber glove on her head?

My mum is with us and she comes into the room.

Thomas, what is your mother doing?

Oh don't worry, Thomas says. Mummy is just looking for our baby.

Silly me. How careless to mislay a baby in the Midwest of America.

Estimates of how long we're going to have to stay in America are constantly changing. Maybe two weeks, maybe three months. It just isn't possible to say. It all depends on the paperwork – getting a US birth certificate for Hope, an American passport, then a British passport. The latter will be the most difficult. British passports in America are issued by the Embassy in Washington, then sent to London and back again. No one knows how long that will take.

Leaving aside the expense, I don't know how we're actually going to make this work. Thomas needs to be at school and we could leave him behind in England for a week or two – but not longer. I realise that I'm facing a situation where one of my children will be in America and one will be on the other side of the Atlantic – with no way of bringing the two together.

Stephen is doubtful as to whether Thomas should go to

343

America. I speak to him. Perhaps you should stay home with Grandma Jan?

No, no, he says. I've got to go to America. I've got to go.

Why?

Thomas looks at me as though I'm stupid.

Because I've got to look after my baby sister. If I'm not there how will I know if she's all right?

And so it is decided that he's coming with us for three weeks at least.

We have lawyers in America, a lawyer in England and a barrister. Now it emerges that we need yet another lawyer, someone who deals with immigration. Natalie puts us in touch with Wesley Gryk and Stephen and I go to see him in London. I expect plush lawyer offices but we find Mr Gryk next to Waterloo Station and he isn't trying to impress anyone.

We are pointed towards a narrow staircase. On a half landing a cramped kitchen opens onto a fire escape, a blank wall. Photocopiers flash in cramped corridors, a water cooler burbles, fans and air conditioning units whirr. A Babel's Tower of languages rises around us. People with turbans, saris, black skullcaps stand in every available space.

Mr Gryk's office is a goldfish bowl with a low ceiling, the windows lined with crooked Venetian blinds. It's so close to Waterloo Station that you can see trains approaching the station at one window and arriving at the other. The walls are lined by bookshelves, with thank you cards propped against them. Fat blue files are piled everywhere. The buildings opposite are stained red brick. A window is open – trains squeal and an orchestra of sirens, traffic and roadworks plays out of tune.

Mr Gryk is tall and thin with close-cropped salt and pepper hair, square glasses with black rims. It is impossible to place his nationality. He appears nervous but explains clearly the various options. We are a textbook case, apparently.

The question is whether we want to try to get a British passport for Hope before we come back to the UK. That takes time but it is more secure. Otherwise we bring her in on a US visitor's visa, but that's risky because she isn't visiting. Stephen and I have already decided that we're going to wait for a British passport.

How long will it take? I ask.

Mr Gryk admits that it just isn't possible to know. But he has contacts in the Washington Embassy. He will be sure to move everything along as quickly as he can. I'm grateful for that but I also know that when a British official decides to leave something in the bottom of an in-tray then it can be there a long time. La-la-la-la. I trust Mr Gryk but he can only do so much. Towards the close of our conversation, he admits that he was the man who got Elton John's baby into England.

I load a short story into the dishwasher, hang Thomas on the clothes line, shout at the washing machine to take its dirty rugby shorts off the stair rail. Now. Right now. The world is a cut-glass chandelier hanging from a frayed rope. At any moment, the rope might break and then everything will drop, smash into a thousand pieces. I take Thomas for a walk on the Common and lose him. One moment he's beside me and the next moment he has gone. I assume that he's run ahead to his friend's house and so I hurry on, calling out his name.

But then I think that I have left him behind and head back. I know that he has been abducted, murdered. And there I am like a trapped ant, under a white sky, up on the lidded roof of the Common, back and forth, hither and thither, yelling and hollering. Finally I stand still, scream until my throat is sand-paper, weep.

When I finally find him he clings to me, his hands pulling tight around me. He was here all the time, he says. Just here. He's shaking, wracked by sobs. I know that it isn't being lost which has frightened him. We sit on the Common together and I apologise to him.

We are into the last month now. Our bags are packed in the hall. Amanda gets in touch to say that, if Hope doesn't come before, then the hospital have scheduled an induction for Sunday 9th October. So the date is set and we plan to fly on 7th October. To me this sounds too late. Don't we need to be there earlier? Stephen says we need time afterwards, not before.

But, of course, Hope may come early. Thomas did. And so we wake every morning not knowing if this might be the day when we have to leave. Secretly Stephen and I wouldn't mind if we missed the birth. It may be six years since Laura died, but neither of us ever want to go into a hospital delivery room again. However, IARC have warned us that if we aren't there within forty-eight hours then Hope will be handed over to American Social Services and this will cause endless legal difficulties.

So Stephen walks around with his passport in his pocket. The plan is that, if we get the call, he'll drive straight to Heathrow and board the first plane. I'll follow with Thomas and Lin as soon as I can. The days are jittery, hysterical. I can't breathe properly. Everything exhausts me. I have to do things very slowly and burst into tears over nothing. I have a headache every day and am missing several layers of skin.

Increasingly my main concern is that by the time Hope is born, I won't be in a fit state to look after her.

Once again we discuss names. Hope was only ever meant to be a nickname. Until now Thomas has been pushing for Arabella Isabella Fenella Kinsella. Stephen and I decide on Isolde. We announce this to Thomas but he's having none of it.

No. No. No. She's called Hope. You can't change her name.

After he's gone to bed, Stephen and I consider this. We're both worried that the name Hope might burden our daughter with an obligation to tell a story which she may consider to be private.

Finally it doesn't matter what we think. Thomas has decided. And we do all like the name Hope. She can have Isolde as a second name. And we'll ask Elena if Hope can have her name as well. Hope Elena Isolde Kinsella. A bit of a mouthful – but a name that contains more than one narrative.

I keep myself calm by making an album of photographs and messages for Amanda and Manda. They know little about us and where we are from, they are unaware of all the family and friends who are excited and grateful for what they are doing for us. I want them to feel a little of that gratitude and also to have a picture of the world which will become Hope's home. Then if Amanda ever worries about Hope, she can open the album and know that Hope is safe and happy, loved.

In general, I consider scrapbooks as an activity best suited to the under tens. But right now it's a good way for me to get through the day. The album becomes an obsession. I surf the internet looking at scrapbooks, choose glues, stickers, ribbons, stamps and papers.

I print off maps of America and England, draw a line of arrows between Marshall and Stroud. I contact everyone who knows about Hope and ask them for contributions. I fill up the pages with photos and messages. People are good at offering messages of welcome to Hope but what I really want are messages of thanks for Amanda. No one mentions her.

I say to Stephen – Maybe they think she's a semi-literate woman locked in a cellar and forced to become pregnant against her will?

Stephen suggests that I need to be forgiving.

We are all in foreign territory here, he says.

As I paste glue onto the back of a photo, position it between lines of ribbon, I ask myself why I am doing this. Is it only for Amanda? Of course not. I'm also keeping copies of all the photographs and messages for Hope herself. Laying a trail for her – a path of gingerbread leading through the forest.

And I imagine how, one day, when she's older, we'll get the box down from the attic and she'll find there all the legal documents, all the photographs, the whole story of her birth. Of course, she may never want to know but it's important to lay the trail. Finding a path back through the past can be important.

I go to see Joslin at the hospice again. The day is not a day for dying. The sun is bright and the fields yellow with cut corn – the one dazzling light meeting with the other, the colours mixing, reflecting, merging. And the land around is burnt dry and dusty, the road to Hereford white as a bone.

I find Joslin faded and flakey like ash. Her thin fuzz of hair has gone grey. She's an image on a white sheet of paper – an image that is being gradually rubbed out, so that finally her whiteness will fade into the whiteness around her and she will be gone. A crisis erupts just as I arrive. A bereavement social worker has just told Joslin that she has between two and four weeks to live. Joslin is furious – How dare that woman be so negative? How can she leave me with so little hope?

Once again the question of the custody of the children is under discussion. Lawyers, wills, divorces, custody. Joslin needs to make phone calls so I sit out on her balcony. Bird food is spread across the balcony but no birds come. The day has become swollen and nightmarish, tinged with green, hysterical, nauseous.

When Joslin finishes her calls, I go back into her room.

I need your help, she says.

Then she tells me to go to the wardrobe and get out a cotton bag that is hidden at the bottom. I get the bag and bring it to her. It is stuffed full of money, stacks and stacks of banknotes, more money than I've ever seen.

There should be £23,000, she says. But I need to count it.

Some of this money has been given by friends. But Joslin also admits that she has been getting small amounts of money out of the bank every month and hiding it under her bed. She's done this because she wants to be sure that the children get some money after she's gone.

Joslin, I say. You shouldn't have kept that much cash in your house.

Yeah, I know, she says. But if someone had stolen that money then they probably needed it more than me – and so then it's OK for them to have it.

All reserve has gone between us now.

You know that's why you're dying, I say. You know that, don't you?

She nods and shrugs. We set out to count the money but the

afternoon air clings and I can't concentrate. My fingers don't work properly. I lose count again and again. Finally Joslin suggests we try another approach. So we work out how thick a stack of £1,000 notes should be and then we measure the other stacks against it. Finally £23,000 seems like a good estimate.

After that the solicitor comes with the new will and we sign that. Joslin is tired and sinks back against the pillows, wincing with pain. She wants me to go, so I kiss her goodbye and tell her that I love her. Then I help the solicitor to carry her bags, and the money, to her car.

This puts me in a difficult position, the solicitor says. You see, I have to account for where all this money came from.

I run through the options in my head hastily.

Oh that's easy, I say. You know Joslin has a great many friends and they've raised money for her. So that's where the money is from. Charitable donations.

The solicitor nods her head firmly. Good, she says. Good. That's helpful. I'm glad you told me that. Of course, that's where it is from.

I put the money into the boot of the solicitor's car and we say goodbye. Then I drive home along the white dust road, through the parched fields. I turn the music up loud and put my foot down hard. My teeth are clenched tight, my eyes watering from the dust. I know that I won't see Joslin alive again.

XXVII

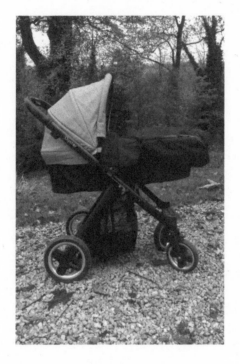

Let us try what love will do.

William Penn

Whenever I'm not making the album, I'm writing. Laying the past out in lines of black and white, neat and tidy. I'm writing to keep sane, to keep the details of the world around me tethered in their proper place. Writing towards Hope, towards the future. Writing it all down so that I can say to her later – this is how it was. Words of apology, of justification or love? Or simply the process of bearing witness, of seeing it as it is.

Joslin dies at the beginning of September, just a month before we are due to leave for the States. I write this down because it is fact, but the truth is that I've never believed it. I went to the funeral, I laid my hand on her wicker coffin, I saw the slides of her artwork at the party afterwards, talked to friends of hers from Glasgow whom I had heard all about but never met. Arrangements were made – Joslin's ex-husband's amazing sister and her husband, who live down in Devon, offered to take Ellie and James as their children, in addition to their own teenage boys. It was decided that Lily would stay in Hay-on-Wye with Wayland and Matthew.

I was told all this, but strangely I remember few of the details. Perhaps the truth is that I simply had to cut off. It had become too difficult to deal with so much life and death. My only comfort is that I know that, if I ever had to explain this to Joslin, she would understand and forgive. I also decided not to be upset that Joslin and Hope could never meet. I feel quite sure that somewhere in the revolving door between life and death, they passed each other, measured the significance of their proximity. Perhaps if the soul really does break down into thousands of pieces which scatter everywhere then some tiny part of Joslin lives on in the baby whom she believed in absolutely and so longed to see. I loved Joslin and I failed her. She gave me so much.

One day to go. Lin arrives, having driven from France via the Portsmouth ferry. Her silver sports car scrunches to a halt on the gravel. The door opens and those long, tanned legs appear. She brings with her foie gras, walnuts and cheese from the Gers. Immediately she makes our trip look like a glamorous holiday.

She takes charge of preparations and everything is suddenly simple. There's really very little we actually need, she says. Together we assemble powdered milk, cot sheets, clothes for Hope. Later we go and pick Thomas up from school and he falls for Lin straightaway. She's going to be good for card games, Sudoku, sweets.

The next morning the alarm wakes us at four. We stumble around in the hall, checking through the bags again and again. Among the many things I've packed are my photographs of Laura. She'll be with us all the way. At the last minute, I wake Thomas and bundle him into his clothes.

Long way to go for a holiday, the taxi driver says.

I decide not to explain. Lin and I sit in the ramrod front seats. As the taxi turns at the end of the lane and sets out across the Common, the wide sky appears, speckled with stars. We pass the turning to Minchinhampton, gather speed as we head towards Cirencester, leave behind the known world.

At Heathrow the man at the check-in looks at the empty pram.

So where's the baby?

Stephen says – We're going to get her.

Really? That's great.

From there we fly eight hours to Newark and then spend three hours in dazzling waiting rooms before the flight to Minneapolis. Lin and I try to order some salad for ourselves and pizza for Thomas, but the lady at the counter doesn't understand. I'd forgotten how foreign America is. After we've eaten, we wander on through the airport, sleepy, disconnected. Everything is too loud and bright. The air is stale and fizzes with an energyless buzz.

Who is the stroller for? a man asks, as he checks our tickets.

Stephen tells him and he says – Wow, no kidding?

The plane from Newark to Minnesota is an airborne sewing machine that rattles us through bright evening sunlight. We sit with our knees under our chins. The seats are brutally upright and my eyes are running because I'm so tired. I look down and see a landscape of grey and khaki. I can pick out a river and maybe houses but one colour merges into another. Thomas is determined to stay awake all the way so that he can tell his friends that he's stayed up twenty-four hours and Lin heroically takes an interest in his Sudoku.

We arrive in Minneapolis and pick up a hire car the size of a small house. When Thomas sees the dashboard, which has dials and knobs like a space rocket, he's jumping up and down with excitement. I sit in the front with Stephen so I can navigate and help to keep him awake. The day is waning but a large sun still flaunts its bronze light. We glide along vast roads, lined by towering, office buildings with mirror windows which flash orange and silver and gold.

Miraculously, we find the road we need with ease and roll away from the city. Everything is big – the road, the cars, the sky. The buildings we pass are long and flat. The light is failing now and I'm struggling to keep awake. Thomas and Lin have fallen asleep on the back seat.

I've seen too many films that start like this, Stephen says.

You know – where the normal family set off for a weekend trip in the wilderness?

The road is long and straight, black and silver, stretching forward into nothing. Darkness falls and we stare into the mesmeric flash of other headlights. Occasionally we glimpse a church, or a traditional white clapboard homestead, surrounded by barns. The signs say: Gaylord, population 2,300; Norwood Young America, population 555; Fairfax, population 1,293.

Only the looping neon lights stretched across the front of diners, or an occasional house with lighted windows, suggest that this land is inhabited. My head nods, then I wake, jerk upright again, talk to Stephen about nothing. Lights wander, winking, through the sky. UFOs, corn circles, alien landings – all seem possible. I call Amanda but she doesn't answer so I leave a message.

The journey is taking far longer than expected. I follow the map, identifying each settlement we pass, but it seems to take an hour for us to move half an inch. We pass through Sleepy Eye, population 1,450. A Road Closed sign appears out of the darkness and we take a turning south. I'm no longer sure where we are. Maybe we should just pull into one of the gloomy motels and stop until morning?

But all the places we pass look like the Bates Motel. In my mind, rocking chairs creak and shadows appear on shower curtains. Ahead of us, a storm is shattering the sky. Flashes of jagged light break across the darkness. Occasionally an explosion of brightness turns the whole sky salmon pink. In those moments of exposure, I look for lights, a town, but see nothing.

My head nods, jerks, nods. I dream of a world in layers like a Russian doll. First a layer of darkness, then a layer of lights, which is Marshall. And then within Marshall a street, and within the street Amanda's house, and inside the house Amanda, sleeping, and inside Amanda, a sealed amniotic sac – containing Hope. Is she sleeping too? Does she hear the storm? Not too far to go now. Stephen sits beside me, his hands gripped on the steering wheel, eyes peering, face white, pressing us on into the darkness.

A road junction, a scattering of lights – apparently we have arrived in Marshall. The sign for the Losada Hotel is straight ahead of us. Modern, functional and low-lying, it sinks into a sea of car park. It looks more like the Middle East than the Midwest. As we pull up, gum-chewing teenagers loiter in tracksuits. Two men stand at a bar wearing cowboy boots and Stetsons. The reception area is Soviet shades of brown and beige. I am reminded of youth hostels I stayed in during my gap year.

Loud music sounds from a cavernous function room. Balloons and streamers are draped around the door. We are told that a college volleyball tournament is taking place at the university across the way. Our room is in Block D, which is so far from the reception that we have to drive to find it. I step out of the car into a night of sticky, tropical warmth. I thought it was meant to be cold here. My bag is stuffed with jumpers and wool tights.

Stephen, Lin and I start unloading the luggage while Thomas sleeps. It seems like a week since we left home. We carry our bags past vending machines, up a lino staircase and along a brown corridor that recedes into the far distance. The rooms are vast with two beds in each, but the ceilings are low and everything is patterned brown. From somewhere loud music throbs and the air conditioning buzzes.

I'm losing my nerve. Our great adventure has become grubby and I want to go home. From downstairs I hear Thomas wailing. I run down the stairs, pull open the car door and cuddle him against me. Mummy, I don't know what's going on, he says. And I don't know where we are. I don't know either but I hold him tight and tell him that everything is fine, even though it clearly isn't. Upstairs I bundle him into bed and drop to sleep myself.

Next morning jet lag wakes us at 5.30. I get up and pull back the net curtains that line the metal-framed window. Outside I see grey drizzle, miles of car park, and a straight line of silver road. Trucks steam along this road, as long as train carriages. It feels as though this is a place of continual motion, everything moving on. Beyond the road is a spaceship industrial plant and, behind that, row upon row of damp, nodding corn.

Thomas and Lin go swimming and I call Amanda. We arrange to meet for lunch at a restaurant called The Hitching Post. I try to unpack our bags and tidy the room but I drop everything I pick up, stumble over the desk chair, knock the kettle to the floor. Thomas and I sit on the bed playing cards until it is time to leave. We are occupying a No Man's Land between the bizarre and the mundane.

Again we are on long straight roads with signs we don't understand. Everything is insubstantial. As soon as we go, they'll pack up the film set and move on. Stores the size of office blocks sell endless sit-on mowers. *What can wash away my sins? Nothing but the blood of Jesus.* We see no people, only cars, sky and distant horizons. Everything here is long, low and flat – the land, the sky, the roads, the trucks, the buildings.

Thomas says – England would fit into one of those fields.

Like everything else here, The Hitching Post is surrounded by miles of car park. Opposite, across a hundred-yard-wide road is a Walmart, a petrol station and offices, all surrounded by miles of tarmac. The Hitching Post is a new building which has the temporary look of a shed or barn. Outside it is decorated with baskets of pink flowers and fake beams. Inside it's all four-foot TV screens and cowboy kitsch: Stetson hats, farm implements, whips, antlers, cowboy boots. And also evidence of hard winters: wooden skis, ice picks, sledges. A notice says – No Dancing on the Tables While Wearing Spurs.

It seems that Amanda and Manda aren't here yet – but would I recognise them if they were? We are shown to a school-canteen-type table. I have presents with me and the album. Every few minutes I get up and walk to the door, then move from one window to the next. We know that Manda worked a night shift so that probably explains the delay. What will I say to Amanda? What will it feel like to hug her when she's got our baby inside her?

Time passes. We order food for Thomas as he is hungry. I go back and forth to the door. Of course, all of this is a hoax. Amanda doesn't exist, the e-mails were all fake. There never was any baby. As we speak, IARC are packing up their sham offices, shredding documents, loading computers and phones into the back of a van. Our money has gone into a bank account that will never be traced. In other areas of America, other duped couples are sitting waiting at diner tables.

And then I turn around and they are there – Amanda and Manda. But Amanda isn't pregnant, she can't be because she doesn't have a bump. So this is the hoax, I think. But still we're greeting them like old friends. I know, Amanda says, I know what you're thinking. Everyone keeps saying it to me – are you sure that's a full-term pregnancy? I hug Amanda and we both laugh as I feel her against me. She's wearing a yellow-and-white-striped top which is stretched lightly over her – or is it our – surprisingly small bump.

My thought is – they're so young, too young to be doing this.

359

Amanda is pale and wears her shining, light brown hair pulled back from her face. Her eyes are large behind thin-framed, oval glasses. Her skin is baby-clear and she wears no make-up. Superficially she appears dreamy, disconnected, but when she looks at me directly I see that she is certain, unshakeable, very young and very sure. And proud as well of what she's done. I am amazed and charmed by her.

Manda is different – short and solid with close cut dark hair, she has the same clear skin as Amanda. But there is nothing dreamy about her. Instead she's vividly present, engaged. Her bright blue eyes are direct and intelligent, and they contain a spark of her humour that lights again and again. She is strong, practical, the kind of woman who could change a wheel on your car. She's protective of Amanda and sometimes speaks for her in a way that is full of love.

They tell us that they met at Walmart. They were both working there. There was three feet of snow and the town was mostly shut down. They were the only two people at work.

They break off, laughing, smiles flash between them like electricity. We order lunch. I keep waiting for the moment of difficulty, the fork in the road, but it never comes. Thomas and Manda are immediately friends because Manda is interested in cars and Thomas wants to know about all the new makes he has seen – their power, the details of their engines and tyres. Also Amanda and Manda have dogs who are called Boston and Brooklyn, and Manda shows him pictures on her phone.

I ask them about the weather, tell them about my bags of wool jumpers.

Yeah, this weather is completely untypical, they say. It's been an Indian summer. The winter could come in any time and when it does the snowdrifts can be as high as the power lines and people can't get out of their houses for weeks.

Manda tells us that Amanda has a talent for funny voices. She's been reading out our e-mails to Hope in an English accent, hoping that when she arrives she'll cry with an English-sounding cry. It's clear that between the Amandas and IARC we've been the butt of a few jokes but we don't mind. Amanda tells us that Hope is very active but she doesn't kick – instead she swoops and dives.

It's as though, for the last nine months, we've been trying to do a jigsaw, but we could never make it work because we only had half the pieces. Now Amanda and Manda have turned up with all the missing bits and the jigsaw falls into place, the full picture emerges. I'd assumed that because surrogacy is more common in America than in England then Amanda and Manda would have found it easier to talk about it than we have. But it turns out that they've never met anyone involved in surrogacy. Surrogacy may be a known path in some areas of America but in Marshall it's still big news.

Amanda and Manda talk about all the excitement felt by their family and friends. Manda is one of five and they are all excited about Hope. It is extraordinary to realise how many people are awaiting her arrival, how many people are part of her story. There is a brief moment when I feel left out. What part do I have in all this? I'm not pregnant, I'm not Hope's genetic mother. Why does anyone need me? But the feeling goes as soon as it comes.

People do get confused, Amanda says. So we have to finish up explaining it again and again. No, she isn't our baby. No, we don't want to keep her.

To be honest, we're looking forward to going home without her, Manda says. Leaving you guys with the diapers and the sleepless nights. It's such a big responsibility. Like, you know, apparently it's really bad for a pregnant woman to fill up at the gas station because of the fumes. And I wouldn't want that for my child and so I didn't want it for Hope either. So I never let Amanda fill up the car.

I'm so touched by this that I find myself close to tears.

Manda tells us a little more about how they came to be interested in surrogacy. We were lying there one night and talking about how sad it was not to be able to have a child, she says. And then I said – but we could do. And so we began to look into all the options. And in doing that we realised that we weren't ready for our own child and we also found out about surrogacy.

I ask Amanda what she's intending to do afterwards. Will you go away for a few days? Take some holiday?

Cherryade Coke, she says. For the caffeine. I haven't had anything like that for ten months.

Amanda and Manda tell us that there is little to do in Marshall. All anyone does is go to Walmart. And because we need to get a few things, and so do they, we decide we'll all go there together. Even though we can see the Walmart, we drive over, following Manda and Amanda. Stephen has some difficulties with the car. Sometimes we can't get the door to open and we can't change the position of the wing mirrors. I ask Manda if she can help.

Sorry. First I ask your partner to have a baby for me and now I want you to be a car mechanic. For a moment I wonder if I've said the wrong thing, but then we all laugh and Manda shows Stephen and Thomas how to work the wing mirrors. Thomas is fascinated by her, sensing that she shares his need to know how things work.

In Walmart everything is huge and shining. The fabric conditioners take up a whole long aisle, the washing powders another. I wander around, lost and amazed. We buy things we need for Hope, and Manda and Amanda come with us, discussing which wipes will have the least chemicals in them, what brand of nappies – or diapers – will be best. I wonder if we are being tactless but Amanda and Manda seem happy. They want to get a camera as well and so we help them to choose.

Finally we part. We will meet again the next morning at six at the hospital and Amanda will be induced then. We head back to the hotel and I'm suddenly overtaken by tiredness and drop into a deep sleep even though we're only halfway through the afternoon.

The next morning we are awake at 4.30, jet-lagged and nervous. An hour later Stephen and I drive down a long straight road lined by burger bars and bowling alleys heading towards the hospital. A mother of pearl dawn spreads across the sky. The hospital is long and low and built of yellow stone with windows like TV screens. It is surrounded by the normal acres of car park. Once again, the weather is oddly warm.

As Stephen eases our bus-like car into a parking space, we see Amanda and Manda heading towards the doors of the hospital. Manda has worked a night shift and is still in her security guard uniform. The hospital seems deserted. Inside, the long corridors are all blonde wood with low ceilings, pale marbled walls. We go to the delivery room with Amanda and Manda. Then a nurse shows us our room: a normal hospital room with a bed and a bathroom.

Our room is some distance from the delivery room, in a parallel corridor. We sit down to wait. I write, Stephen reads an English newspaper left over from Friday. After an hour or so Manda comes to find us and asks if we want to see Amanda now that she has changed into her hospital gown. We find her propped up in bed with monitors attached.

I'll probably sleep quite a bit, she says. People don't believe that I slept through labour when I was having Olivia, but I did.

You do whatever you want, I say. And have any drugs you want.

I don't think I'll need anything, Amanda says. Although maybe this time I will, since I'm being induced.

We can hear the heartbeat on the monitor and it booms at us with a rhythm that makes us all want to dance. Not surprising, Manda says. We know Hope is a dancer. We chat a little longer and then go back to our room. When I pop in again later, Manda is sitting beside a big pot of moisturiser that she's using to massage Amanda's feet.

Maybe this single-sex relationship thing is a good idea, I say to Stephen.

A nurse overhears me and says – Just what I was thinking. If I come back for another life, I think I'll go that way. Because, I tell you, we have a lot of men in this hospital and I've never seen any of them massaging their wives' feet with moisturiser.

At nine o'clock the hospital cafeteria opens and so Stephen and I go and have breakfast. The canteen lady asks where we are from and I tell her about Hope. She wears a white cap and a hairnet. Now she's smiling so widely that her eyes are all creased up. I promise to let her know when Hope arrives. Then I eat bacon and sausages and hash browns. It seems terrible to be sitting eating while Amanda is in labour upstairs but I'm starving.

Manda pops down to tell us that Amanda's waters have broken. She's nervous but I'm not and I don't know why. I'm calmer than I might be on any day at home. All this seems quite mundane, just a baby being born. We meet Dr Hartfiel, the doctor who is going to deliver Hope. She tells us that she deliberately scheduled the induction for a Sunday so all the staff would have plenty of time. I'm suddenly glad that we are going through this strange process in Marshall, because it is a place full of small-town slowness, small-town kindness.

Then the door opens and a man walks in. He's medium height, middle-aged, casually dressed. His hair is strawberry blonde and cut close to his head. He's talking but I can't understand what he's saying. Then I get it. I'm afraid that something has gone wrong. I'm really sorry that I have to tell you – We've lost the baby.

But he isn't saying that at all, instead he's talking about politics. I read his name badge: Dr James Hanna. I don't really understand where he fits into all this, but he's telling us that he tunes into those parts of the BBC that are available in America. The current economic policy in Britain is a terrible mistake.

I leave Stephen talking to Dr Hanna and walk around to see Amanda and Manda, but the door is shut and a nurse tells me that they are both asleep. I get talking to the nurse, tell her that I'm worried about not being worried.

Well, one way or the other, she says, I wouldn't worry now. You've got the next eighteen years to do that.

I go out for a walk. It's a glowing autumn afternoon, the trees are pale gold and they spread their colour to everything around them. The hospital is in a residential area and around it there are streets of single-storey clapboard houses, widely spaced, arranged along roads with those green signposts which are so familiar to me from films.

I am wearing too many clothes and am hot. Everywhere seems strangely deserted. Squirrels hop along the pavements and the occasional American flag waves on a front lawn. On the drives there are RVs the size of double-decker buses.

Golden leaves drift down through the silent air. I catch glimpses of other people's lives – net curtains, mailboxes, sandpits in the garden, cane chairs on verandas, spider plants hanging in baskets, television screens flickering.

Later, I fall asleep on the hospital bed with my cardigan spread over me. I don't know how I can sleep but I do. Nurses called Janel and Jen keep popping by with news. They are waiting for Amanda to be four centimetres dilated. That's when active labour starts. She's nearly there now, they tell us. And still hoping not to have an epidural, but let's see how it goes.

I lie curled up on the bed, waiting. Jen comes in and says that maybe Hope might be born after another couple of hours. Stephen is still reading the newspaper. It's around five o'clock and outside the light is seeping from the day. The view from the window is onto a courtyard. In the distance we can see the windows of the cafeteria where we ate earlier.

Then Jen comes in and says that Hope is coming. I thought we still had two hours. Stephen and I don't know what to do. We always said that we wouldn't be there for the birth, but we want to give Amanda all the support we can. Jen ushers us around to Amanda's room. The door is closed and we wait. Tears are flooding down my face and I'm struggling for breath. A nurse finds a chair for me. Stephen and I are arguing. We can't change our minds now, he says. But I know that Amanda wants us in there.

This is getting quite real now, he says.

Shut up.

Dr Hartfiel comes hurrying up the corridor.

Are you guys coming to cut the cord? she says. But still we hesitate.

Once in a lifetime experience, she says, and disappears into the room. We hear a muffled cry and then another. The door is opened and we're pulled into the crowded space. I'm pushed towards Amanda's feet. I lock my hands over my face and sob, because I can't draw breath. Two nurses are holding me up. My mind is clouded, my body flooded with terror.

You can look, the nurses say. You can look.

I open my fingers a crack, see white flesh stained with a flash of red and something like a rope, pale yellow and shining. I press my hands over my eyes again. I can't hear any more cries and I can't see Hope. She must be dead. Someone is telling Stephen where to cut.

I'm pushed to where a plastic tray is lined with sheets. And then suddenly Hope is there. She's bright red and screaming, her legs kicking, her tiny arms waving. They lay her in the plastic cradle and start to clean her up. I want to pick her up, I need to pick her up. She's screaming and screaming, and her solid small arms and legs are thrashing through the air.

I stroke her head, take hold of her tiny, wizened hands. She's alive, very definitely alive, more alive than anyone I've ever seen before. Dark red and perfect. I long for the doctors to stop doing whatever they're doing. Hope is in a storming rage. I'm in floods of tears and look up and see Manda across from me and she's crying as well.

Finally they wrap Hope in a sheet and guide me to a sofa in the corner of the room. Then they pass her to me and I feel her tiny weight in my arms. She's screaming and screaming but I don't mind at all. I'm happy for her to keep on screaming for as long as she wants because that's how I know she's alive.

For a long time, I sit on that sofa holding Hope. Stephen goes to fetch Lin and Thomas. As soon as Thomas arrives he wants to hold his sister and so we sit him on the sofa and put her on his knee. I ask if Amanda wants to hold Hope but she says that she'd rather not as she's still in pain. One of the nurses finds a Cherryade Coke for Amanda.

Later, Stephen takes Thomas and Lin back to the hotel again so that Thomas can go to bed. Then Manda's family turn up – her mother, stepfather, her younger brother and younger sister. After a while Amanda takes a turn at holding Hope, but I notice that she keeps her at arm's length. Quite soon she hands her back because she's still tired.

Manda's stepfather wears a baseball cap and a T-shirt which says America – Land Of The Brave. Initially, he stands in the doorway looking awkward but gradually he is drawn into the room.

So what kind of roof does your house have?

Uuum?

Roof.

Oh right. Yes.

I remember that he's in the roofing business. So I tell him that our roof is pretty rare: Cotswold stone slates, which should last for hundreds of years, which is good news because they are incredibly expensive to replace. Then I tell him about the restoration of our house, all the work that had to be done on the guttering, the problem of the hidden gullies in the roof which must be cleaned out regularly. And then we go on to other roofs. Fortunately, everyone in my family lives in an old house that they have renovated so I'm quite good at roofs.

Gradually, I understand that this is a big stretch for this baseball-capped man. Like some of our elderly relatives, he is lost in this world. His stepdaughter is in a single-sex relationship and her partner has had a surrogate baby. I tell him about my mother's roof, the problem with the lead gullies that are not deep enough. It's just the level of rainfall now, that's the problem, we agree. At least you know where you are with roofs.

And there I am. It's nearly midnight, and I'm in a town in America that I've never visited before, a place which may not actually exist. And I'm in a room full of strangers talking about roof tiles. But I have never been so happy in my life because Hope is lying in my arms and she is all that I need.

XXVIII

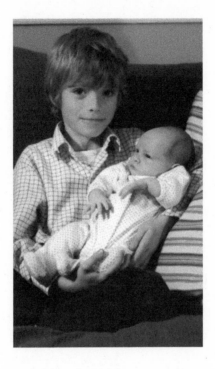

Every baby born into the world comes
with the message that God is not
yet tired of mankind.

Rabindranath Tagore

We spend the next three days at the hospital with Amanda, Manda and Hope. From the beginning, we take care of Hope. The staff move an extra bed into our room, and Lin and I sleep there with her beside us in a hospital cradle. Everyone comes by to see us: the CEO of the hospital, doctors, the kindly dinner lady. A nurse arrives with a hand-knitted hat and blanket for Hope. Apparently every baby born in Marshall Hospital is given these gifts and they're knitted by ladies in the town.

The air is muggy and we eat too much. Sitting on the bed in our room, we pass Hope between us, cuddle and feed her. Lin takes charge of the bottles and I'm grateful for that as I'm so fuzzy headed that I can't remember how that works. We expect the hospital to get busier when the weekend is past, but it never does and consequently everyone we deal with works with a reassuring slowness, takes time to chat and answer questions.

Amanda is up on her feet again immediately after the birth. She looks like she's just come back from holiday. She clearly likes to look at Hope but has made a decision not to hold her. She tells us she wants to pump milk for Hope and, remembering how much I hated pumping milk myself, I'm amazed and grateful. She wants Hope to have the best, she says.

Is Amanda OK? We ask Manda again and again.

Manda assures us that Amanda is fine, although sometimes even she isn't sure.

She did look down at her stomach, Manda says. And it's all hanging loose in folds. And she seemed kind of sad then. But I wasn't sure whether she didn't like Hope's absence, or whether she was shocked at the state of her stomach muscles. I think it was the latter.

During those days in the hospital, life stories are exchanged and more pieces of the jigsaw are slotted into place. Thomas talks to Manda endlessly about cars and does monkey impersonations for the nurses. As far as he's concerned, this whole surrogacy business is great because you get masses of time off school. He takes photographs of everything – even the loo – so that he will be able to describe it all to Hope when she's older. He does like to look at Hope but he bursts into tears every time she cries.

One afternoon I find myself alone with Manda and we talk about her relationship with Amanda. Marshall, Minnesota sure is a conservative place, she says. It's not easy being in a single-sex relationship here. Some people are disapproving. Others seem to think that we're some kind of adult movie. Either way the attention can be unwelcome. Even some of my own family find it pretty difficult.

It occurs to me that some of Amanda and Manda's quiet confidence comes from their sexuality. I've seen this in other gay people. They have a strange, unswerving certainty precisely because they haven't been able to rely, as so many of us do, on outside approval. They've had to learn to approve of themselves, no matter what anyone else thinks. Maybe it is also this certainty that has given Amanda the courage to be a surrogate mum.

Amanda has loved carrying Hope, Manda says. And you know what? She's already thinking of doing another surrogacy. She's told the agency that she needs a little bit of time off, but in a few months she'll be ready to work with another family.

There are times, during those long, breathless days at the hospital, when I long to be left alone. Some small part of me wants to pick up Hope and say – She's mine and I don't want to share her. But then I remind myself that I will have her for the next eighteen years and longer, and so I can easily share her for a few days. And all of these people have helped to make her, have cared for her and worried about her. They've given Amanda the support she needed to carry Hope.

Sometimes when I pick Hope up I feel her tiny head pressing against me, her lips reaching out towards my breast. When that happens, tears spring to my eyes because I feel bad that I can't breastfeed her. But I have so many other things to feel happy about that I'm not going to let this one disappointment spoil my happiness. There are many ways to be a good mother and breastfeeding is only one of them.

On the evening of the third day, it's time for us to leave the hospital. Amanda and Manda are leaving as well. I have dreaded this moment, even though I know that this certainly won't be the last time we'll see the Amandas. We all feel as though we've been in the hospital for weeks, and now we're not sure how we'll cope in the real world.

For Stephen and me, this moment brings back the horror of leaving the hospital without Laura. He says – Do you think any other couple have left three maternity hospitals under three such different circumstances? But those other hospital departures are now the past and this time we're going home with a baby brimming full of life.

We say goodbye to Dr Hartfiel. She's a brisk and practical woman, not given to displays of emotion, but she knows that our thanks are sincere. Stephen and I know how carefully she orchestrated our situation, how fully she had briefed her staff.

As with so many other aspects of this situation, I admire the American talent for doing a job properly. Nothing is random, nothing is left to chance.

We also say goodbye to Jen and Janel and Dr Hanna, even though we'll be coming back to see him again so that Hope can have a check-up. Then we all head off to the lifts together and walk out of the hospital, gasping. And there I am, out in the fresh air with the rows of clapboard houses stretching away from us.

I'm soaked in tears, hug Amanda and say yet again – Are you OK?

Yes, she says. I'm fine. And she gives me her open, quizzical smile and shrugs her shoulders, pats me kindly on the arm. And then finally I understand. I see the truth. Some women are born to do this. Their role is to carry a baby in love and then to hand it over to another woman graciously and without any questions asked. This is their vocation, their role in life. These women exist – and twenty-nine-year-old Amanda from Marshall, Minnesota is one of them.

Two days later, we go to court. Steve Snyder is driving from Minneapolis, and Amanda and Manda will be there as well. The court is behind Main Street, which looks exactly like an Edward Hopper painting – low rise with blinds hanging out over all the shops, the road running wide and straight in between. The warm weather has gone and winter is sharpening its knife. Hope is asleep in her Maxi-Cosi, wearing a little cream wool hat that Lin knitted for her. The courthouse is a featureless red-brick building. The lady at the reception admires Hope.

So who is the mother? she asks.

I hesitate, but Amanda is quick on the draw.

She is, she says, pointing at me. I wonder if I should explain that Amanda is the one who did the hard work, but this lady just wants to admire Hope, she doesn't need the whole story.

None of us knows what to expect.

Maybe we'll find out we got a parking fine, Stephen says.

Other than the lady at the desk, no one else seems to be around. I have the impression they've opened up the building just for us. Steve Snyder is delayed by the same road diversion that delayed us six days ago. Eventually he arrives. He's less formal than I expected. A stocky man with grey spiky hair, humorous and efficient. He tells us that all we have to do in the courtroom is agree with what he says.

We are called. The courtroom has no windows and half of it is filled with white plastic chairs. The other end has the judge's bench, which is semicircular and made out of dark wood. Altogether there's as much brown and beige here as at the Losada Hotel. A vast American flag with an eagle on the top is propped into a metal stand. There's no one in the courtroom except a lady sitting beside the bench, writing in a book, and a policeman.

Steve, Stephen, Amanda and I sit on chairs to the side of the bench. The judge enters. All stand. Amanda is asked to stand up, raise her hand and promise to speak the truth so-help-me-God. Then Stephen has to do the same. I am irrelevant in this process. We are here to take Amanda's name off the birth certificate and confirm Stephen as Hope's father. As a result of this process, Hope will finish up with a birth certificate which carries Stephen's name but has no details of her mother. Isn't it usually the other way around? Apparently this is what we need for the moment.

In the introduction Steve refers to Elena as the genetic mother and presents papers that state that she has given up any right to Hope. I find this a little awkward. We haven't spoken much to the Amandas about Elena. In a way, Elena's contribution to this process is more important than Amanda's, but still Amanda carried Hope for nine months and went through the labour. Documents are presented from Dr Yatsenko in California explaining the medical procedure involved.

Steve begins by questioning Amanda. Is it correct that you entered into this agreement? Did anyone force you to sign it? Steve goes through the whole story from the beginning. Amanda is calm and answers again and again. Yes, correct. Yes, correct. She's warned that if she gives up her parental rights then she'll never be able to recover them. She's told that, although she might have made a private arrangement with us to keep in touch, this has no force in law. She's asked how much she was paid.

Twenty thousand dollars.

Then Amanda is asked intrusive questions about how she knows that Hope is the result of the medical transfer in California. She's asked – Could this be your child? She says that theoretically Hope could be her child but practically she couldn't. She's asked to clarify. I'm gay, she says. So she isn't mine.

I want to protest about these questions but Amanda never flinches. Then it's Stephen's turn. I promise to speak the truth so-help-me-God. Again Steve goes through every detail of the arrangements we've made. Stephen answers. Yes, yes. That is correct. I find it strange to see him in the witness box. The hunter hunted. Steve only falters when he has to state where we were married – Worcestershire. And where we live now – Gloucestershire. Steve points out that we've waived our right to a paternity test. He asks if we feel sure that Hope is our child.

She looks like her brother, Stephen says.

You're aware, the judge says, that clinics can make mistakes and that, if this has happened, then in law you still remain the father of this child.

I look at Hope and wonder. What if there was a mistake? But I don't care. Hope is our child and we're taking her home. Sleeping in her Maxi-Cosi, Hope fills a nappy loudly and smiles in her sleep, her little cream hat falling down over her eyes.

It's clear that the judge has probably never dealt with a case of this kind before and is relying on Steve. Normally the court decrees that a period of time should pass before decisions are made, so that anyone can change their minds, but the judge agrees to waive the normal procedure so we can get back to England in a reasonable timescale. The lady taking notes is from Social Services and she's asked if she has anything to contribute but she doesn't. The judge states that she's satisfied and that the new birth certificate will be issued.

All stand. Then the judge comes over to congratulate us and takes a look at Hope. Manda, Thomas and Lin come to join us. Thomas points out to the judge a couple of spelling mistakes in the documentation and coaches her in the correct pronunciation of Worcestershire and Gloucestershire. I thank Amanda for all that she has done. You were great as well, I say to Manda.

Yeah, she says. No one holds a chair to the floor as well as I do.

Then it's all over and we're leaving the court. We arrange to meet Manda and Amanda later. It occurs to me that when we leave they might miss Thomas more than they miss Hope. Hope has slept straight through her legal transfer from Amanda to us, her lips pouting contentedly, her tiny hand gripped around the edge of her blanket.

When we get back to the hotel, I phone Mum. She has just

been to see the premiere of my new play and she tells me that everything went well. I feel as though she's reporting news from the moon.

Later, I sit down at my computer and send an e-mail message to everyone we know announcing Hope's birth. I don't hold back on the details and record our thanks to Amanda. As I'm going down the e-mail list, I come to Joslin's name. I feel as though I should e-mail her. Maybe she still picks up messages wherever she is?

Immediately messages from friends come back. All are enthusiastic, kind. My father even manages a one-line e-mail, which is more than I expected. One message says – You have bent destiny to your own purposes. I try this version of events on, as one tries on a new dress, and briefly I feel bold and powerful. But finally this isn't the look for me. I am unconvinced. We go back to being people who have engaged in something rather underhand.

Some messages are typed by people clearly in shock. After all, there are people who know us well who were told nothing about the surrogacy. I read through the messages again, find them evasive. Everyone seems keen to welcome Hope but no one says much about Amanda. What I really want is for people to ask how they can thank her for what's she done. I say this to Stephen.

Yeah, he says. But it's normal. I mean, Hallmark don't have a card for it, do they? Marriages, seventieth birthdays, even death. But there's no card which says Congratulations on your Egg Donor and Surrogate Birth, is there?

I decide to take Hope out for a walk. I want her to have her first proper outing in the fresh air and I need exercise, solitude. The hospital air was muggy and the hotel isn't much better. Also, I want to give Lin a break because she's been with us all the way, dealing with all the difficult baby stuff. We could never have done this without her.

And so I set off, walking down the side of the road with the pram, as there are no pavements. Despite the width of the roads, the cars which come past slow right down and swing out wide. And the drivers stare at me – friendly but puzzled. I don't think that they see any women walking with prams here. I walk for two hours and never see anyone else doing the same.

I come back along long streets of clapboard houses. Outside nearly every house there are pumpkins despite the fact that it's still three weeks to Hallowe'en. One house is draped with the Stars and Stripes. *Support our troops, keep America safe.* The clapboard houses are drowsy in the afternoon heat. Hope is only half asleep, her eyes watching the light shifting above her. It's no longer just a case of NRTIHRN. Something Really Wonderful Is Happening Right Now. I'll never be much happier than I am in this moment – just walking with my daughter in the afternoon sun of this alien, welcoming town.

We spend the next few days exploring Marshall. Sometimes Amanda and Manda are with us, sometimes not. We find a coffee shop which sells something approaching a European coffee. This is a great relief. Stephen and Lin had been threatening to drive three hours back to Minneapolis for a coffee. In the evenings, we sometimes go bowling with the Amandas.

Later we have dinner and discuss breast milk. I'm beginning to worry about this question. The issue is – should Amanda stop pumping when we leave Marshall or could she continue? Elton John set the bar high by having breast milk sent by Fedex to England. And it's clear that anybody who is anybody in the world of celebrity surrogacy does the same. But the medical profession don't actual agree that this procedure is safe. The milk needs to be kept frozen and Fedex don't guarantee to do this. Amanda says in her easy-going way that she's quite happy to stop whenever, but it's clear that she's researched the Fedex option. We agree that it seems criminal to throw the breast milk away, but apparently donating it to a hospital is not an option. You have to go through loads of medical tests before you do that to ensure you don't transmit an infection.

My feeling is that Amanda should stop pumping so that she can get her life back, but maybe I'm once again making assumptions about what Amanda wants. The question is left unresolved but I feel that we've at least put down a marker that maybe we don't want Amanda to continue for much longer. But still I'm worried. Everything has gone so smoothly and I dread causing offence over this most emotional of issues.

That night I have a bad dream. Hope has been split up into several pieces – she's white and flaky, like pieces of bread spread on a lake to feed ducks or fish. But all the bits of her are breaking up, dissolving into the water, spreading far and wide. And somehow I have to gather them back together. I have to scoop the bits of my baby out of the lake and make her whole, gather her to me and make sure that no part of her drifts away.

We've been in Marshall ten days now and it's time for us to leave. We have no choice because, now the new birth certificate has been issued, we have to apply for a US passport and we can only do that in Minneapolis. We spend our last morning at the Losada packing up. I'm still worried about the breast milk situation. Thomas bounces up and down on the bed and sings – We're leaving the brown hotel today, hoorah, hoorah.

Once we've packed up, we go meet the Amandas for lunch and suddenly the breast milk issue is settled. The Amandas are coming to Minneapolis on Saturday for a surrogate social organised by IARC. Amanda will wind down the pumping and bring whatever she pumps to Minneapolis with her. As ever, it's Amanda who has navigated a route through these tender waters.

What's a surrogate social? Thomas asks.

Amanda explains that it is a party which IARC organise every year for all the surrogates who work with them. This year the party will have a Hallowe'en theme. Stephen immediately asks if he can come along, but the Amandas tell him it's not for Intended Parents, only for surrogates. Stephen feigns offence, continues to plead until they tell him to shut up.

We pay the bill and step outside into a freezing wind that tugs at coats, hair, scarves, the doors of cars. Winter is definitely on its way and, now that I've felt the edge of that wind, I'm not so sure that I want to experience it. It's so cold that our goodbyes are hurried. We all agree that we'll reschedule the crying until we say goodbye finally in Minneapolis. Then we set off on the three-hour drive to Minneapolis. This time we can see the countryside. It rolls past us, unchanging.

The corn is all taken in now so the fields are naked and pale yellow. Farms have Dutch barns and big silver grain storage units with pointed roofs. The sky is burnished pink and grey-white, and stretches away all around to endless horizons. Power lines loop low over the land. Vesta, population 319. Redwood Falls, population 5,254. We're on the road home.

XXIX

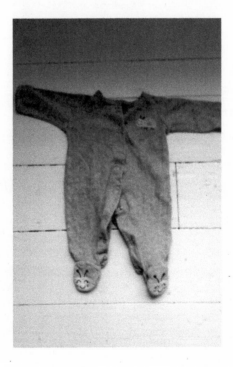

Live, then, and be happy, beloved children of my heart, and never forget, that until the day when God will deign to reveal the future to man, all human wisdom is contained in these two words, 'Wait and Hope.'

Alexandre Dumas – *The Count of Monte Cristo*

Minneapolis is a massive road junction lined by fast-food restaurants and factories. We stay at the Homewood Suites, 1500 Wayzata Boulevard. Our apartment is on the seventh floor and has two bedrooms and a sitting room with a galley kitchen. It's brown – but a better class of brown. The windows don't open and air conditioning whirrs. A ten-lane highway passes silently below. The city centre is visible across the urban sprawl, a science-fiction cluster of glistening mirrored skyscrapers rising up through the hazy, car-fume air.

We all get up early that first morning and head to Maple Grove, the suburb where IARC's offices are located. We've been in regular communication with IARC for two years but I've no idea what their offices look like. It turns out they're in a business park which looks like a residential development of white clapboard houses. Their offices are far smaller than expected and feel like a private house or an upmarket doctor's surgery, all dark wood and oriental carpets.

We meet all the staff we've e-mailed so often over the last two years. Keely hands me a package that has been sent by Elena. I open it to find two little babygrows. They are blue and grey with plenty of poppers and will cover Hope from head to toe. I am impressed. This is the kind of present a real mother gives, a woman who has brought up triplets. No bows or ribbons, no cute pale colours which will be ruined in weeks. Once again I feel some strange affinity with this woman I have never met.

While I continue to chat to Keely, Stephen disappears to speak to one of the lawyers. Forms have to be filled out for copies of the new US birth certificate, and the US passport application has to be completed. So far it seems that the legal process is developing as it should, but Stephen is checking every detail. The American lawyers find it hard to understand why the law in England is different to the law in America. Their silent question is – If this works for the States then why doesn't it work for you? This has been the eternal problem of what we're trying to do. Two legal systems need to be meshed together but they're completely different and were never designed to work in tandem.

Now Stephen calls Wesley Gryk in England, sitting atop Waterloo Station, to check whether the new birth certificate needs a stamp or not. He trusts IARC and knows that they are doing their best, but they struggle to understand how pedantic UK officials can be. If there's one tiny mistake on the UK passport application then we could all be in the States for weeks longer than planned. I'm grateful that Stephen is dealing with all of this.

Saturday afternoon arrives and the Amandas find us at the Homewood Suites. They arrive with pots of breast milk for Hope, the last that she will have. They've just been to the IARC Hallowe'en surrogate social. Stephen is longing to hear about it.

Presumably the women who are pregnant go as pumpkins? he says.

Amanda says – No, but there was one woman dressed as a positive pregnancy test stick. You know, all in white with a red line across her middle?

Apparently Steve Snyder went as Indiana Jones with a long whip curled at his waist. We can none of us work out where this fits in with the Hallowe'en theme, but agree that Steve is clearly the Indiana Jones of the surrogacy world.

Stephen, Thomas and the Amandas start playing Uno and the conversation turns to Elena. I show the Amandas the babygrows. We haven't talked about her before because it seemed tactless. It can be tricky to manage the demands of competing mothers. Thomas knows about Elena but he likes to pretend he doesn't.

What is this chicken-egg thing? He asks. He always refers to Elena as the Chicken-Egg Lady although I've told him plenty of times that the whole thing has nothing to do with chickens. Now I explain it to him again, as best I can. I know that partly he's showing off, but I need to be gentle because over the last few weeks he's had a crash course in all sorts of new subjects: single-sex relationships, assisted reproduction, genetics.

I would have preferred him to sort out the birds and the bees, I say. Before getting onto the duck-billed platypuses of the reproduction world.

Soon we set out for an early supper at a restaurant across the parking lot. Manda starts a night shift at ten so they'll have to leave by seven. This will be the last dinner. Some tiny part of my mind wants it over with – wants my baby to be mine, wants to cut loose from everyone else's claims on her. But ninety per cent of my mind aches at saying goodbye. Of course, we say we'll be back to visit soon, but will we? The journey is over twenty-four hours.

The time spins out. I get worried that Manda will be late for work. Finally we pay the bill and walk out of the restaurant. Then we cross the car park towards the hotel and their small red car. We shrug and shiver and I hug Thomas. Both of us are close to tears. And then there's nothing else except to say goodbye. The Amandas hug Thomas and then I hug them both.

You changed our lives, I say. And you didn't even know us.

We did it together, Amanda says, and then she shrugs and gives us her easy-going smile. Will we see them again? The truth is that few relationships endure over long distances. Amanda and I were never good at e-mailing. And yet the link will always be there. Whether it's five years, ten, twenty, I feel sure we will meet, and that we'll be able to pick up pretty much where we left off. Who knows what the intervening years will do to us or to the Amandas? I hope that the world will be kind to them. God bless them both. They deserve so much happiness.

As they get into the car and drive off, I hurry back towards the Homewood Suites and Hope. I can't look back but keep on walking through the freezing night air, hugging my arms around myself, warding off an empty feeling of friends made and lost.

On Monday we go with Steve Snyder to the passport office in downtown Minneapolis where we make an application for Hope to have a US passport. Then in the evening Stephen and I go out to dinner with Steve and his wife Christine. We go to a place called Pittsburg Blue Steak in Maple Grove. Inevitably we talk about surrogacy. Steve says – pleasantly – that he considers many Europeans to be hypocrites. There are so many countries where it isn't legal, he says. Spain, Italy, Poland. And yet their businessmen and government ministers, and even the leaders of the Catholic Church, are on my doorstep as soon as infertility strikes in their families.

Is there anyone you won't work for? I ask. He says that generally he leaves those kinds of decisions to the medical profession. They have guidelines from the Human Embryo and Fertility Authority but they don't have to follow them. Before he ran the agency there used to be a rule that both partners had to be under fifty. But, he says, there are people of fifty who are healthier than people in their thirties.

The Indiana Jones of the surrogacy world. To me all this seems worrying. How far do you go? Where do you draw the line? Clearly I have no right to comment, given what we've just done. And there is something refreshing in the American lack of judgement. Steve's attitude is certainly very different from the moral, controlling English, who can always see a problem, even when one doesn't exist.

We talk to Steve about the hierarchy of Hope's various mothers. I have no claim, I say. I have done nothing – but I will do the next eighteen years and more. Probably Elena is most important as she has the genetics, but she's never touched Hope or seen her. And Amanda is important and she isn't.

I don't know, Steve says. In the end, I think you all did it together. If Hope has three mothers then I'm sure that they've all given her something positive.

The days are ticking away now until Stephen and Thomas leave. Thomas has been in the States three weeks and the second half of his school term starts soon. We'd always told him that, no matter what, he'd need to be back home by then. Lin and I will have to stay on until Hope's British passport arrives. This might take a week – or longer, much longer.

I am scared of Heathrow. Hope will have a UK passport and a US passport so she can enter the country legally, but still I dream of some problem with paperwork, some mistake, which means that they'll refuse us entry and put us on a plane back to America. The authorities at Heathrow have been told to look out for surrogate babies and recently a couple were sent back. Another couple were detained for hours and only allowed to enter the country after signing endless papers committing them to regularise their situation immediately.

The last day comes and we set off at midday to pick up

Hope's US passport. We expect a delay but we're in and out within minutes. After that we head to the Water Park of America, which is the biggest covered water park in the States. Everything here is big, bigger, the biggest. Lin and I sit in a vast rubber ring with Thomas and whizz down a helter-skelter type slide which is ten storeys high. Thomas wants to do it again and again and so Lin and I whizz and tumble and splash until we feel sick. Catching Thomas as we drop from the end of a slide into a turquoise pool, I grip his arm tightly, wishing that he could stay.

Stephen and Thomas leave. I stand in the car park, watch them drive off. When I go back to the flat it looks empty without their things. They've also taken the hire car back so we have no transport. The days that follow are quiet, dreamy, stationary. Lin and I feed Hope, chat, go to the supermarket or coffee shop, knit.

One day, I take Hope out for a walk in her pram around the suburban area behind the Homewood Suites. The light is silver and still, blurred by a soft mist. The leaves are mainly down from the trees now, but the occasional flash of yellow or fiery orange still flares among the tangled grey branches. No one is around, the houses are shut up and silent. As in Marshall, they are spacious, detached, white clapboard, but here the ground rises and the gardens are surrounded by woodland.

We pass a yellow school bus standing at the entrance to yet another unending road of shuttered houses. It appears to be empty but, then, as I walk on, I see the driver, grey-grizzled and stooping, standing by the bus staring down the road. I realise then that he has got out of the bus in order to watch as a small boy with a backpack walks away down the narrowing, mist-blurred road. That boy must have been the last child to get off the bus and perhaps he has further to walk than the others before he reaches home?

I don't know. But, for whatever reason, I stand and watch the crumpled old man standing in the suburban road, watching the boy grow small in the distance. Finally the boy, who is now no more than a speck, turns and waves. Clearly he has reached his own home. The man waves back, his bent hand drifting in the air for longer than is really necessary. I want to go and say thank you to the man because he has taken such good care of the small boy.

Of course, I don't actually say anything. But as I turn the pram, ready to set off back to the hotel, I know that that image of the man and the gradually diminishing boy on the mist-silver road is the image that I'll retain long after the other details of these days have blurred.

I start to write again, my laptop propped on a long narrow desk against the window. Below me, traffic on the ten-lane road moves silently by. I get back in e-mail contact with old friends from the Quaker Meeting House in Brussels and remember how patient they were when I had a thousand questions about faith. I still have a few of those questions, but now they are of merely intellectual interest.

I may not believe in God but I do believe in goodness. And I believe in the importance of seeing things exactly as they are, of knowing just how difficult and cruel this world can be. Look that in the face, know it fully, and then get on and enjoy everything you can. That's seems to me to be the way to live.

One day dissolves into the next. It's just the UK passport, that's all we're waiting for now, but we have no idea how long we might have to wait. The passport has to be agreed in

Washington and then forms have to be sent to London, where the passport will be issued. It will then be sent back to us in the States. Wesley Gryk, the UK immigration lawyer, is responsible for this part of the process and he's briefed the Washington Embassy. It shouldn't take too long.

But I lie awake at night worrying. What if the man at the Embassy is on holiday or sick? Or what if the authorities simply decide not to cooperate? Stephen and I haven't broken the law but we have circumvented UK public policy. So far the public authorities have accepted this – but what if our application arrives at the moment when someone decides to object?

A week passes with no news. Stephen and Thomas call us from England. Thomas is back at school and my mum is helping to look after him. On the phone he sounds shaky. I need to get home soon. After I put the phone down, I start to cry. If the passport doesn't come soon then I'm going to have to insist that we take him out of school again, that he flies over to be with me here.

Then, without warning, an e-mail comes to tell us that the UK passport has come. It's at IARC's offices and they offer to send it over. I imagine it lost on one of those wide highways and tell them that we'll come and get it immediately. Lin and I discuss what we should do. Surely we need a day to organise ourselves for the journey? But Stephen calls and tells us he can get us on a flight in the morning and we decide we'll go. Why wait any longer? If we leave now we'll be arriving back in the UK one month to the day after we left. Both Lin and I are dreading the journey, but she's calm, assures me that it'll all be fine. Together we go and collect the passport and say goodbye to everyone at IARC.

The next morning we're ready early, take a cab to the airport, speeding away from Wayzata Boulevard. Will we ever come back to this particular place again? I don't suppose we will. At Newark we have a three-hour wait. As we sit down for a coffee, I open Hope's US passport. I haven't looked at it in detail before. On the inside cover I find an image of a naval battle scene and the words of the US national anthem – *O say does that star-spangled banner yet wave, o'er the land of the free and the home of the brave?* I would once have dismissed those words as sentimental and grandiose, but now I reflect on just how many people in America have been brave for us and am pleased that Hope will always carry a bit of America with her.

After Lin and I have finished our coffee, I pace back and forth through the airport. What if we get turned back or detained at Heathrow? I have Natalie's mobile and contact details for Steve and Wesley. I also have a US and a British passport for Hope. Stephen has also written and signed a letter authorising me to travel with Hope. We know from past experience that we may need this because I do not use his surname.

Surely with all these documents there can't be a problem? I call Stephen to tell him that it looks like the flight will arrive at 07.00 as scheduled. Then I call my mum. She's just been out in the fields with the dogs. Wonderful, she says. Nearly home now. I'll get the kettle on. Godspeed.

The flight to Heathrow is full. Boarding is like a rugby scrum. I'm terrified that someone is going to drop a case on Hope but Lin has got her gripped tight. We ask if we could swap to a seat next to the aisle but this request is refused. We have informed the airline that we're travelling with a month-old baby but no one seems to care.

But Hope falls asleep, and sleeps and sleeps. She's still tiny enough just to fit on Lin's knees, although not mine because my legs aren't so long. She wakes once to feed but then sleeps again. Lin and I look at each other, roll our eyes, wonder how long our luck will hold. On the screens in front of us a diagram shows the plane travelling across the Atlantic. I look at this screen again and again, willing the time to pass. No one from the airline ever asks if we need any help.

Finally the flight comes to an end and Hope is still sleeping. As we leave the plane, Lin complains to the staff about how rude they've been but they don't care. So we head on, pushing Hope in the pram, reclaiming our baggage and heading for the passport queues – which snake for miles around the airport. Lin and I look at each other in shock and hastily join the queue. A lady looks into the pram and then at me.

Oh my, didn't you get your figure back quickly?

The queue is endless – businessmen, Indian families in their traditional dress, mothers with squalling infants, backpackers with tans and mosquito bites. I am more and more nervous. Please, please, don't let us be sent back to America. Finally I make it to the front of the queue and step forward, pushing Hope. The pram is covered by a cotton blanket as we're trying to keep Hope asleep. I hand the passports over and wait for the man at the desk to tell me to remove the blanket but he never does.

Is this your baby?

I consider saying – *How long have you got?*

Instead I say – Yes.

But you don't have the same name.

No. But I have a letter of authorisation from my husband, the baby's father.

I grapple for this letter, hand it over.

Yes, but this doesn't prove anything. What you need is a copy of the baby's birth certificate.

I freeze. I've got so many documents but the only birth certificate I have was issued in the US and doesn't have my name on it. I take a deep breath. The lights are focusing in on me, displaying me to everyone in the airport. An insistent ringing starts in my ears, the arrivals hall has gone strangely silent. I shuffle papers helplessly. The official's eyes are lasering through me. Then suddenly he raises his hand. Is it possible that he won't insist on the birth certificate? That hand hovers in the air for days, weeks, before he waves me on.

And we're home, home, walking towards the exit. Free. Safe. I've never been so glad to feel English soil under my feet. Just three days after this, a government inquiry will be launched into slack immigration procedures at UK airports. We are lucky. I call Stephen to tell him we're through. He says that Thomas has been waiting for the news and that he'll get a message to him at school. Lin and I stumble out through the exit and suddenly my mum is there and I am in her arms. Under the glaring airport lights, she holds me tight. Later she'll tell me that she got up at four, drove to Stroud, found our taxi man, hitched a lift with him to Heathrow. Now she looks down into the pram where Hope still sleeps. Welcome home, my little one.

XXX

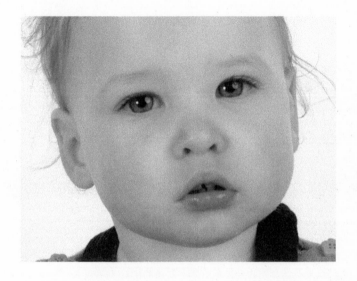

One must still have chaos in oneself to be
able to give birth to a dancing star.

Friedrich Nietzsche

I put the washing machine on, hang clothes on the line, change the cot sheets, write in my diary, wipe Hope's nose, listen to Thomas do his piano practice and complain about problems with the wi-fi. It's three days after our return from America, a bronze-bright evening, surely the last of our Indian summer. Hope is already in bed and Lin and I are making the supper. A knock sounds at the door. Dave, who helps out in the garden, is there with his white van.

Phew, he says. Long day. But there and back all right.

Sorry?

Brussels, he says. Terrifying those tunnels but I managed all right.

What?

The rose bush, he says. Found it OK.

Stephen emerges from his office and I realise that he organised for Dave from Tetbury, who has never driven on a foreign road, to go to Rue du Châtelain 26 and bring home Laura's rose bush. He has it now in the back of his van. Of course, the rose bush might not survive the journey, or the deer in our garden, but at least this little part of Laura has come home to us.

A few days later, Lin and I take Hope to Weston-super-Mare. It's a dishwater day with a tugging wind, but still I take Hope from the pram and walk out with her over the sand, towards the sea, until freezing waves break over my boots. Then I lift her up high so she can look out to sea. She smiles, or I imagine she does, and I think of all the days we'll have together on the beaches of the coming years. Better to focus on that rather than on the fact that I will still be doing the school run when

I'm in my sixties, that I'll hardly have finished claiming child benefit before I get my pension.

When Lin and I get home, my mother has come to tea and she brings a present. As I tear the tissue paper a shiver ripples up my arms. Some part of me already knows. Blue wool appears, a stiffened edge of navy velvet. A coat emerges – velvet-covered buttons, fitted at the waist. Laura's coat. The one I have always imagined. The one she wears as she runs – endlessly – in that frost-glittered garden. But the strange thing is that I have never had any discussion with my mother about that coat. When I mention it now, she understands immediately. She also has always imagined Laura wearing just this coat. Perhaps that isn't really so strange. Many middle-class mothers choose this style of coat for their daughters.

Some part of me wants to stuff the coat away in the back of the wardrobe and leave it there. But why should Hope miss out on her present? Is it not better to welcome the coat as a testament to the unspoken links that exist between mothers and daughters, the mysterious concurrence of imagined worlds?

The question of whether we will bond with Hope never arises. Hope has decided to bond with us and she's not taking no for an answer. Perhaps because she had three mothers, she has the energy and determination of three babies. She can turn her head through three hundred and sixty degrees. People who know nothing about us, and about her history, call her Mrs Happy because she spends all day smiling.

A month after we get home, I'm walking through Stroud and I meet a woman I don't know well. Seeing the pram, her face clouds in a moment of confusion but then she smiles down at Hope, clucks enthusiastically. Of course, she says. I remember. I saw you three months ago, didn't I? And you were heavily pregnant then, weren't you?

She is not the only person to make this mistake. I don't bother to explain.

On another occasion, at the school gate, I overhear someone talking about us.

Yes, incredible, isn't it? They just flew over to America, picked up the baby and that was it.

I tell Stephen about this and he laughs.

Come to think of it, he says. Why didn't we just get her sent by DHL?

It's important to tell your own story, otherwise someone else will tell it for you and they will almost certainly get it wrong.

There is still the issue of the two remaining male embryos in California to be settled. We speak to Dr Yatsenko who tells us we have three choices – the embryos can be destroyed, they can be donated for scientific research or we can pass them on to another couple anonymously.

Could we give them to someone and make ourselves known to them? I ask.

Dr Yatsenko says that this is unusual but possible.

I should warn, he says, that because the embryos have been frozen, the chances they will lead to a successful pregnancy are only 40 per cent.

Yes. But 40 per cent would sound like a pretty good statistic to some couples.

Dr Yatsenko admits that this is true and we promise to call back when we've thought this through. Once again we are back into complicated moral questions. If these embryos are used then Stephen could be a father again, Hope could have a full sibling, or two. Maybe we should keep things simple and just donate the embryos anonymously? But I wanted Hope to have the chance to know her genetic origins so should I now deny that chance to another child?

Stephen and I hesitate. We are both envisaging a moment in twenty years' time when a child, or children, travelling from America turn up on our doorstep wanting to meet their genetic father, and the sister they have heard about. The thought is daunting but the way ahead is clear. So many people were brave for us, now it's our turn to be brave, our turn to pay into the general pot of kindness. We sign the papers and send them off.

And have we become Ambassadors for surrogacy? Not really. Stephen and I have spent long hours since we came back from America talking on the phone to other couples who want to set up surrogacy arrangements in the States. The view that we give them is honest, lacks any element of marketing or persuasion. Surrogacy is a desperate measure, for desperate times. But it can and does work. It saved our lives. And there are women like Amanda who, through their own free choice, want to be surrogate mums. Is it right for any system of law to prevent these women from fulfilling their destiny? Shouldn't our society celebrate their generosity rather than criticise them?

Possible changes to the UK surrogacy laws are debated by the media endlessly. In general, the people who give their opinions have no direct experience of surrogacy. Often they've got the basic facts wrong. It is beyond question that changes do need to be made to the current legal framework in Britain because it is hopelessly outdated. But should surrogacy become easier in the UK? I don't know. Surrogacy is like abortion, mercy killing, prostitution – all of these things will happen anyway so why not create a proper legal framework to safeguard all those involved? There will always be Karen doing DIY in Doncaster so why not bring her under the protection of the law?

And international surrogacy? In reality, the process in America is so different from India or the Ukraine that there is no point is discussing them in the same breath. But one thing is certain – international surrogacy isn't going to go away. The internet and the relative ease of foreign travel mean that people will continue to seek solutions abroad. But, sadly, international surrogacy is far beyond the means of many who desperately need it. I'm conscious – painfully conscious – that our story has a happy ending because we have money. And I know only too well that many women need a baby more than I did. I do not forget those women but I also know that my guilt will not benefit them.

Maybe adoption will become a real option for more couples? Two weeks after we get back from America, a government inquiry finds the UK adoption system 'unfit for purpose'. One hopes that judgement may prompt change, but complaints about the system stretch back over many decades so expectations inevitably are low. Certainly I am left with questions about why we couldn't have given a home to an existing child instead of creating a new one. And some part of me will always be haunted by that baby who we might have adopted – and who is probably still waiting for a family and a home.

When Hope is eight months old, we go to the High Court to apply for a Parental Order – the last leg of the great paperchase. If we achieve this then we'll be issued with a new birth certificate for Hope which will have my name on it. This will mean that she'll be completely and truly mine and that no one will ever be able to challenge that.

Natalie has assured us that all will go well, that there won't be a problem. But I am haunted by the extra money we paid to Amanda, the money which might not be considered 'reasonable expenses'. I know that, whatever happens, Hope is not going to be snatched from my arms. But if something does go wrong then we could be involved in years' more legal hassle, we could even have to go through a whole adoption process. I'm praying for the whole thing to be finished with today. Tomorrow we leave for a holiday in St Ives. Knowing that, one way or another, we'll be at the seaside in twenty-four hours, steadies my nerves a little.

But it isn't only the big issues which worry me. I'm also anxious about taking an eight-month-old baby into the High Court. A social worker will be there and will be commenting on my fitness as a mother. What if Hope screams the place down? What if she has a leaky nappy or smears banana everywhere?

The Leveson Inquiry is taking place at the High Court and a giant plaster model of Rupert Murdoch is mounted on a stick. A young woman with dreadlocks holds a banner saying – News Not Boobs. We fight our way through crowds of photographers. Thomas is wearing a white shirt, school trousers and tie. We've even managed to persuade him to comb his hair.

The entrance to the courts is the size of a football pitch, cavernous, a forest of arched columns, like a church. We meet our social worker, Jane, and also Natalie and our barrister, Ruth. Wigs and gowns scurry back and forth. We're ushered out to the back, where a 1970s building – glass and dark wood – houses the family courts. It still isn't clear which judge we'll have and apparently this does matter. The Honourable

Justice Lucy Theis, who Natalie hopes will hear our case, might be tied up on another matter.

Finally an usher directs us all into the courtroom. It is a windowless room of dark brown wood. The bench is high up and we sit opposite on lower wooden benches. Ruth is at the front, ready to speak on our behalf. Natalie carries numerous lever arch files that contain the submission which has been made on our behalf. The Honourable Justice Lucy Theis arrives. All rise.

Some vital document is missing and she goes again. We wait around. Hope is crawling around on the floor, picking up pieces of dirt and eating them. She's going to be hungry soon and she will need solid food as well as milk. She has always refused to eat anything off a spoon, preferring to take matters in hand herself. Banana could finish up on the ceiling. The judge comes back and questions are asked. It is clear that the judge knows both Ruth and Natalie. They have all worked together before. Stephen, Thomas and the usher are the only men present.

Questions arise about some papers that Amanda hasn't signed. Although in the US court she signed away her rights to Hope, she also needed to sign UK papers as well. Natalie was aware of this but had assured us that it won't matter. And now questions are being asked about 'reasonable expenses'. Hope is burbling and wriggling, getting increasingly raucous and hungry. I put her on the floor and she crawls for a few minutes but then wants to be picked up. I realise that we're not going to get the Order. Some of the paperwork is missing. More questions, more looking at documents.

Then suddenly everything is agreed. The judge gives her judgment and it is recorded. Hope is referred to as being Vocally Present in the court. And then later as Swimming Along The Bench. We have got our Parental Order with only one visit to court. We are the first people ever to do this, a legal precedent. It's publicly recorded that we did everything within the law.

And then suddenly it's all at an end and we are walking out of the court room. I didn't know that I had been horribly stressed by the experience, but I feel like a puppet with its strings cut. Hope is ours, definitely and completely. No one can ever take her away. We walk away together down the London streets, Hope wiping rusk into her silver hair. Stepping forward into normal, into the future.

The next day I'm pushing the pram along the seafront at St Ives, thinking of all that has happened to us over the last seven years. Has the empty chair at our table been filled? No – and it never will be. But, paradoxically, those families who come together at a table where there is an empty chair sit more closely together. They understand the idea of family as fortress. And now that we have Hope, the gap is less obvious.

Some things will never fix. Stephen still has asthma and his balance remains mysteriously poor. I have given up expecting to gain a normal level of manual dexterity. My texts look like Chaucer's English. Thomas knows that he is responsible for threading needles, peeling shell from hard-boiled eggs. He himself worries far too much about whether something bad will happen to Hope. But leaving those aftershocks aside, have I arrived at a place of acceptance? No and I never will. The very word has a deadly ring to it. If I reached that place then I would have stopped caring and I will never do that.

Believe me, it was none of it for the best. I'll keep on raging against the loss of my babies because that way I'll know I'm still alive. All who live should rage. People who are angry get up in the morning, people who are sad sometimes do not.

I did not learn useful lessons or become a stronger person. Those who stress the benefits of suffering have failed to make their case. The existence of darkness has no effect on the brilliance of light. I am still here – that's the most that can be said. But nevertheless it is time, as Joslin said, for the But in the sentence to be changed to And. Time to forgive the Pharisee who had more pressing business and walked on by. Time – finally – for the Spectre to sit down at the Feast.

I walk on, look out across the silver and jade blur of Porthminster beach, wondering at the sheer there-ness of it all. What is it that fascinates me about the sea? Am I just another of those writers for whom it is the most obliging of metaphors? The sea as the subconscious, the ultimate symbol of mystery, of invincible power, of eternity. The sea as an image for the fragility of humanity in the face of the great forces of nature. Blah blah blah.

No. The truth – now that it arrives – is, as always, less grandiose than one expects. It isn't the sea itself that interests me, not really. It's those wind-worried towns clinging to the shoreline and all that they promise. Not genteel St Ives, but those dingier resorts that garland the English coast. Ice cream, fish and chips, donkeys, candy floss. A helter-skelter and a big wheel, sun hats and bare feet, a big dipper and a mini train.

But those towns hardly ever deliver that – or only for a handful of days a year. Instead they are usually places of stinging rain where the sea dashes in, dirty grey and sinister, roaring and bubbling, doubtless full of sewage or detergent. Seaside towns are the ultimate act of defiance. A glorious, determined, reckless celebration of the refusal to accept reality. Yes, there will be ice cream and donkeys, fish and chips and a helter-skelter. We will still dream of good days. And this finally is the metaphor of those towns. The hope, the continuing hope – despite all the evidence – that it will not be so.

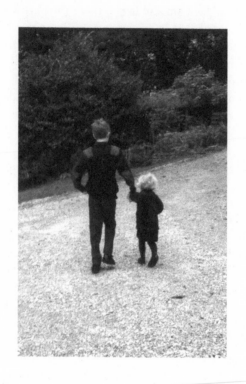

Those seeking further information about some of the issues raised in this book may find the following organisations useful:

Sands (The Stillbirth and Neonatal Death Charity)
www.uk-sands.org

The Donor Conception Network
www.dcnetwork.org

The Miscarriage Association
www.miscarriageassociation.org.uk

Brilliant Beginnings
www.brilliantbeginnings.co.uk

Natalie Gamble Associates
www.nataliegambleassociates.co.uk

The author's proceeds of this book are being donated to
SANDs (The Stillbirth and Neonatal Death Charity)

IN MEMORIAM

For Our Beloved Son, Bradley Allen Engels
– Love, Mom & Dad.

Isabel & William Cansell.

William Michael Simon, 16 December 2010

Nils Verle, 25 May 2008.
Never and forever.
xxx

In ever loving memory of Ainle and Fintan Woodhouse.
Forever in our hearts, you walk with us still.
xxxxxxx

To our loving daughter Lily Rose Irie Iddenten
sadly taken away from us on the 4/10/2007.
Always in our thoughts, missed so much.
xxxx

In memory of our Annie-Rose Jessop.
Twin sister of Daisy-Anne and sister of Charlotte.
xxxx

Matthew 'Pip' Richardson – 24th July, 2003

In memory of our beautiful twins,
Laura Catherine Aandahl (29.10.2003–06.11.2003) and
Lucas Alexander Aandahl (29.10.2003–13.11.2003)

In memory of Conrad L. Wace, 1962–2011.
Loved and remembered every day.

Madison Jessica Cox
My beautiful angel born sleeping on the 07/08/2014

Martha Tillie Bullock – 20 May 2005

In memory of Lucy Sutcliffe, stillborn on 28 April 2003,
whose little life had such a big impact;
heartbreakingly sad, but so positive too.

Ella May White: 24th December 2014 – 6th January 2015

In memory of my baby son, Matthew James.
Love you always, darling. x x

In memory of Jonathon Laurence Fox (18/02/94 – 20/02/94)
twin brother of Lachlan, brother of James and son of
Linda and Chris. Loved and missed forever.

To my babies, Ollie George, Emily May and my other
precious baby, I will always love and remember you.
Shine bright little ones.
Mummy x x x

IN MEMORIAM

James Antony Parker: 22.09.2013

In memory of Seth Stanley Davis
who was stillborn at 40 weeks on the 1st May 2013.
Brother to Isaac, Orli & Jemima.

In memory of Eleanor 24/06/2000.
'In memory of those taken too soon, all you have to
do is look at the moon, you'll find the brightest
shining star and they won't seem so far.'
Always in our hearts never far from our thoughts.
xxxxxx

Precious memories of my baby son Christopher Eric
who was stillborn on 21 February 1983.
When I should have said Hello, I had to say Goodbye.
xxx

17.11.11
Our combined love created you, all our hopes and dreams
in a parcel, forever cradled in our thoughts.
Chloe & Yvonne. xxx

Angela Felicity Peters. 28th August 1991 – 21 January 1993.
'There isn't enough darkness in the world to extinguish
the light from one small candle.'

Thomas Edward Dimbleby,
26th November 1975

Bradley Allen Engels,
Our Beloved Son.

Gabriel Holloway Hellens stillborn 30.11.95.
Loved and missed every day.

In loving memory of babies Molly Traynor (14.04.11)
& Grace Traynor (04.05.12)

Woodlet Wilson,
daughter of Michael and Sam, always in all our hearts.

It's an honour to support this.
Chris Watson.

For our beautiful angel
James Antony Parker 22.09.2013

Victor.

Nicola Pettifar,
6 Sept. 1960 – 12 Dec. 1960

SUBSCRIBERS

Dear Reader,

The book you are holding came about in a rather different way to most others. It was funded directly by readers through a new website: Unbound.

Unbound is the creation of three writers. We started the company because we believed there had to be a better deal for both writers and readers. On the Unbound website, authors share the ideas for the books they want to write directly with readers. If enough of you support the book by pledging for it in advance, we produce a beautifully bound special subscribers' edition and distribute a regular edition and e-book wherever books are sold, in shops and online.

This new way of publishing is actually a very old idea (Samuel Johnson funded his dictionary this way). We're just using the internet to build each writer a network of patrons. Here, at the back of this book, you'll find the names of all the people who made it happen.

Publishing in this way means readers are no longer just passive consumers of the books they buy, and authors are free to write the books they really want. They get a much fairer return too – half the profits their books generate, rather than a tiny percentage of the cover price.

If you're not yet a subscriber, we hope that you'll want to join our publishing revolution and have your name listed in one of our books in the future. To get you started, here is a £5 discount on your first pledge. Just visit unbound.com, make your pledge and type **dbst** in the promo code box when you check out.

Thank you for your support,

Dan, Justin and John
Founders, Unbound

Unbound is a new kind of publishing house. Our books are funded directly by readers. This was a very popular idea during the late eighteenth and early nineteenth centuries. Now we have revived it for the internet age. It allows authors to write the books they really want to write and readers to support the writing they would most like to see published.

The names listed below are of readers who have pledged their support and made this book happen. If you'd like to join them, visit: www.unbound.com.

Rebecca Abrams
Jules Acton
Denyse Molaro Adamson
Sultana Afdhal
Zareen Ahmed
Jane Aitken
Clare Algar
Helen Ali
Danish Ali
Giampi Alhadeff
Clare Andrews
Nick Andrews
Rosie Arkwright
Sandra Ashenford
Dr R V Bailey
Kim Baker
Deanna Bates
Sally Bayley
Anna Beer
Christine Bell
Jo Bloom
Isabelle Bonnard

Clarissa Botsford
Wayland Boulanger
Vanessa Bowcock
John Boyce
John Boyle
Lorraine Blencoe
Jo Bradshaw
Sherry Brennan
Andy Brereton
Rose Bretécher
Ben Brown
Miranda Bruce-Mitford
Sarah Buckingham
Linda Bullock
Marcus Butcher
Ruth Cabeza
Isla Campbell
Una Campbell
Jill Cansell
Xander Cansell
Kate Carpenter
Louise Cartledge

Mary Cavanagh
Sarah Spencer Chapman
Amal Chatterjee
Chloe & Yvonne
David Clasen
Vanessa Cobb
Malinda Coleman
Rachel Connor
Jeannette Cook
Elly Cooper
Isabel Costello
Madison Jessica Cox
Helen Craig
Sue crawford
Hannah Cullen
Richard Curnow
Sue Curran
Christopher Curtis
Ed Read Cutting
Alex Dampney
Judith and Geoff Dance
Louise Davis
Jody Day
Mieke Debrock
Jo Derrick
Michael Dickson
Sian Digby
Harrison Jack Donkin
Philip Douch
Jenny Doughty
Jane Draycott
Elspeth Drayson
Anne Drew

Danielle Dummett
Carrie Dunham-LaGree
Clare Dunkel
Gillian Eastwood
Vincent Eaton
Hattie Edmonds
Jude Emmet
Amanda Faber
Alison Falconer
Katie Fforde
Andrew Fielding
Pauline Camacho Fielding
Angela Findlay
Liz Flanagan
Janet Flight
Caroline Foster
Isobel Frankish
Jan Frazer
Nadia French
Naomi Frisby
Helen Froggatt
Lauren Fulbright
Phil Gaskell
Kim George
Julia Gilbert
Cherry Gilchrist
Purusha Gordon
Rebecca Gould
A.J. Grace-Smith
Voula Grand
Wesley Gryk
Sarah Green
Lucy & Sylvain Guenot

Lorna Guinness
Sam Guglani
Nicki Hales
Claire Hannah-Russell
Linda Hepper
Shahla Haque
Simon Hargreaves
Maire Harrington
Mary-Anne Harrington
Felicity Harris
Lindis Harris
Nicky Harrison
Caitlin Harvey
Kate Havrlik
Haynes Family
Clair Hector
Anne Hemsley
Anthony Hentschel
Victoria Hobbs
Jessica Hodge
Gillian Hodson
Heather Hodson
Lindsay Pilbeam
Lisa Holden
Abigail Holloway Hellens
Kate Holmden
Amanda Holmes Duffy
Antonia Honeywell
Clare Hudman
Lucienne Hughes
Sabrina Hunt
Anna James
John James

Katie Jarvis
Jeremy Jennings
Louise Cogan Jennings
Andrew Johnson
Jan Jolly
Victoria Jolly
Kathleen Jones
Kyra Karmiloff
Elena Kaufman
Barbara Keenan
Rachael Kenningham
Dan Kieran
Alice King
Carla Kingham
Mike and Micheline Kingston
Alice Kinsella
Andy Kinsella
Angela Kinsella
Jo Kinsella
Laura Kinsella Foundation
Marian Kinsella
Stephen Kinsella
Laura Kirk
Paula Kneen
Susan Knox
Caz Knight
Mary Laws
Deborah Lee
Marti Leimbach
Adam Lent
Jacqui Lofthouse
Siobhan Loftus
Virna Lorenzon

Nikki Love
Sally Lovell
Jo Lowde
Gail Haslam Loose
Maurits Lugard
Jane Mace
Katherine MacInnes
Lin Mackinnon
Shona Main
Kate Mallinckrodt
Marc Mangoni
Maya Matthews
Philip McCauley
Robert McLeod
David Melvin
Maarten and Rosário
Meulenbelt-Dias Diogo
Annabel Mills
Martin Mills
John Mitchinson
Bel Mooney
Clare Morgan
Harriet Moynihan
Frederick Mulder
Hannah Mulder
Catherine Naughton
Matthew Newman
Jamie Nuttgens
Rebecca O Donnell
Joanna & Charlie O'Malley
One Fine Stay
Emily Palmer
Deborah Parker

Anna Patient
Poppy Peacock
Tim Pears
Alison Percival
Simon Pettifar
Nicola Phillimore
Robert Phillips
Lindsay Pilbeam
Irene Pinner
Justin Pollard
Craig Pouncey
Permille Pouncey
Emma Pouncey
Saskia Pouncey
Gill Powell
Belinda Pyke
Lotte Quinn
Katie and Jools Randall-Stratton
Griet Randolph
Alison Ravano
Natasha Rawdon-Rego
Imelda (Mel) Read
Andrea Rees
Julia Rees
Kay Reid
Christobel Robertson
Cari Rosen
Caroline Rowland
Jan Royall
Rebecca Rue
Jane Rusbridge
Daisy Susan Hannah-Russell
Richard and Helen Salsbury

Caroline Sanderson

Anna Sathiah

Paola Schweitzer

Stephanie Scott

Rosalind Scrutton

Holly Shaw

Sonal Shenai

Amanda Sheppard

Audley Sheppard

Sarah Shilson

William Simon

Jules Skelding

Lynda Smith

Arthur Snell

Steve Spinks

Tom Squire

Clive Stafford Smith

Pam Stanier

Loretta Stanley

Gillian Stern

Raoul Stewardson

Catherine Stewart

Anne Summerfield

Katie Sutcliffe

Emma Sweeney

Helen Taylor

Edwina Thomas

Jackie Thomas

Carla Thompson

Elizabeth Thompson

Sam Thompson

Sara Thornton

Rebecca Topping

Peter Touche

Helena Townley

Claire Traynor

Marianne Valmens

Kerri Vermeylen

Katie Waldegrave

Meg Walker

Belinda Walthew

Miranda Ward

Sharon Waring

Melissa Watkins

Caroline Watson

Martin Westlake

Alison White

Liz and Martin Whiteside

Joanna Whittington

Naomi Wildey

Miranda Williams

David Wood

Mary Rose Wood

Ainle Fintan Leslie Woodhouse

Victoria Woodhall

Anuita Woodhull

Shirley Woolner

Peter Wragg

Zhanna Zhaksybek

Meike Ziervogel

A NOTE ABOUT THE TYPEFACES

Jan Tschichold (1902–1974) was a German calligrapher, typographer, book designer, teacher and writer. This book has been typeset using a digital representation of his design, namely, Linotype Sabon.

Sabon-Antiqua, designed by Jan Tschichold for both hand- and machine-composition, was issued simultaneously by the Linotype, Monotype and Stempel type foundries in 1967. The designs for the roman were based on the type designs of Claude Garamond (c.1480–1561) and the italics of those by Garamond's contemporary, Robert Granjon.

The chapter figures are MB Empire Heavy, designed by Ben Mecke Burford at M-B Creative, UK.